A synopsis of
CHEST DISEASES

A synopsis of
CHEST DISEASES

JOHN COLLINS
MD MRCP
Consultant Physician, Brompton Hospital

BRISTOL
JOHN WRIGHT & SONS LTD

ISBN 0 7236 0526 2

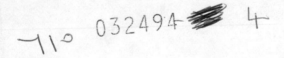

710 032494 4

Printed in Great Britain by Billings & Sons Ltd., Guildford, London and Worcester.

To Helen, who never counts the cost.

PREFACE

My primary aim in writing this book is to provide for medical students a simple but comprehensive account of the common chest diseases encountered in the United Kingdom. I hope that it may also prove useful to graduates preparing for the MRCP and as an occasional source of reference to the general physician. Because there are already many excellent accounts of pulmonary physiology and its applications to clinical medicine, I have kept these sections small but a list of useful references is given at the end.

I am very grateful to a number of my colleagues and friends who have read parts of the text covering their own fields of interest but I must be held entirely responsible for any residual errors of fact or bias. Such thanks are due to Drs Peter Cole, Duncan Geddes, Margaret Hodson, Dai Jones, David Mitchell, Glyn Morgan, Anthony Newman-Taylor, Ian Petherham and Charles Turton.

Thanks are also due to my friend Robert Kirkman for the design of the illustrations and to Miss Catherine Read and Miss Janice Clarkson who typed the many drafts and corrections to the manuscript with unfailing patience.

Bernard Lucas and Don Emerson were enthusiastically supportive while I was writing and Mr Adrian Symons of John Wright & Sons Ltd kindly carried me through to publication. To them I offer thanks although they are in part to blame for encouraging me in the first place. Helen, Jonathan and Phillipa have never complained when my attention has been distracted by the urge to write, perhaps they were sustained by the hope that it would get it off my chest!

London, 1979   John Collins

CONTENTS

THE HISTORY

INTRODUCTION

The diagnosis and treatment of respiratory diseases are based upon a thorough history with special reference to cough, sputum, haemoptysis, breathlessness, wheeze and chest pain, together with attention to details of past history, previous treatment, family and social history, occupational history and details of previous chest X-rays. The outline to be followed is:

1. Details and duration of major symptoms.
2. Time and mode of onset of first symptoms.
3. The pattern of development of further symptoms.
4. The progress of the illness and related disability.

SYMPTOMS OF RESPIRATORY DISEASE

Shortness of Breath. Breathlessness or dyspnoea, although a subjective phenomenon, can often be described in detail by the patient with help from the physician. The following features should be sought:

1. Character: Rapid shallow breathing (tachypnoea) which occurs with pulmonary oedema or anaemia may be differentiated from the wheezy expiratory breathlessness of asthma, bronchitis and other causes of expiratory airways obstruction.

2. Circumstances: Its relationship to exercise, meals, posture and time of day.

ORTHOPNOEA or breathlessness lying down, a symptom of heart failure, may also be caused by pressure of the abdominal contents against the diaphragm in patients with lung disease.

PAROXYSMAL NOCTURNAL DYSPNOEA. This is another symptom of heart failure and it may be confused with paroxysms of breathlessness and cough at night in patients with asthma and less often with chronic bronchitis. Careful attention to details of the history and examination will usually allow a distinction to be made between heart disease and these other diseases. An electrocardiogram, spirometry and a search for eosinophilia may be needed.

STRIDOR due to inspiratory obstruction may be recognized by its loudness and timing.

BREATHLESSNESS OF SUDDEN ONSET. This may occur in pulmonary oedema, pulmonary embolism, pneumothorax, acute asthma and inhalation of foreign bodies.

BREATHLESSNESS OF GRADUAL ONSET. A common feature of chronic bronchitis and fibrosing lung disease.

GRADING BREATHLESSNESS. It is helpful to grade breathlessness on exercise as for example:

1

Grade 1 – Able to walk with family or friends on the flat but at a
reduced pace.

Grade 2 – Has to slow or stop when walking on the flat alone.

Grade 3 – Breathless on dressing, washing and walking about the
house.

Grade 4 – Breathless at rest.

Cough. Breathlessness and cough are the commonest respiratory symptoms.
Cough is a reflex response to irritation of receptors lying within the
mucous membrane and is designed to clear excess secretions from the
airways. Cough of recent onset is common with upper respiratory tract
infections, acute bronchitis and pneumonia and occasionally a spontaneous
pneumothorax. Left ventricular failure may also present as paroxysmal
cough.

PERSISTENT COUGH. Chronic bronchitis is the commonest cause of
persistent cough but affected patients do not often complain of it.
Other causes include bronchial carcinoma, bronchiectasis, tuberculosis and, rarely, benign endobronchial tumours. Recurrent
paroxysmal cough in the early hours of the morning is a feature of
asthma. Persistent, irritating cough without other symptoms often
follows uncomplicated respiratory tract infections.

COUGH SYNCOPE. In paroxysms of coughing, transient loss of consciousness from cerebral hypoxaemia may result from impairment
of cerebral blood flow due to the sustained increase in intrathoracic
pressure with coughing which prevents adequate cardiac output.

SPUTUM. Only produced if bronchial secretions are excessive.

Mucoid Sputum. Common in asthma and non-infected chronic
bronchitis.

Purulent Sputum. Yellow or green in colour, is usual in acute or
chronic bronchitis, bronchiectasis, cystic fibrosis and lung
abscess. In asthma eosinophils in the sputum may give a spurious
appearance of purulence.

Frothy Sputum. Tinged with blood, is produced with frank pulmonary oedema.

Black or Grey Sputum. May be produced by town dwellers due to
the inclusion of carbon and dust particles in mucus. Sputum
production exceeding 50 ml per day suggests the presence of
chronic bronchitis, bronchiectasis or cystic fibrosis. If it is foul
smelling, suspect bronchiectasis and infection with anaerobic
organisms.

Haemoptysis. Haemoptysis or bloodstained sputum must be differentiated from haematemesis and staining of saliva by blood from
the mouth or nose. Copious haemoptysis can occur with bronchiectasis but otherwise the quantity of blood produced is not
helpful in establishing the cause.

Causes of haemoptysis include:

1. Bronchial tumours, especially carcinoma.
2. Pulmonary infarction.
3. Pulmonary tuberculosis.
4. Acute pneumonia. In pneumococcal pneumonia the sputum usually has a rusty tinge.
5. Bronchiectasis.
6. Lung abscess.
7. Mitral stenosis. Haemoptysis may be caused by pulmonary oedema, bronchial infection and pulmonary emboli.
8. Pulmonary oedema with and without heart failure.
9. Chronic bronchitis.
10. Trauma, including lung contusion.
11. Coagulation abnormalities.
12. Goodpasture's syndrome.

Chest Pain. As with all pains the following features are important: mode of onset, character, site, radiation, duration, intensity, precipitating, aggravating and relieving factors.

1. PLEURITIC PAIN. Typically sharp, worse on inspiration and coughing, and may be referred to the shoulder tip. Common causes include pulmonary infection or infarction, malignant disease, tuberculosis and spontaneous pneumothorax.
2. TRACHEAL PAIN. Presents as retrosternal soreness, worse with coughing and is common in acute tracheitis.
3. CHEST WALL PAIN. Severe pain made worse by movement and local pressure, is a feature of rib fractures, erosion of ribs and intercostal nerves by neoplastic disease, but is most often caused by musculoskeletal injury from persistent coughing.
4. ILL-DEFINED CHEST PAIN. Causes to be considered include carcinoma of the bronchus and mediastinal involvement by tumour or other processes. Myocardial ischaemia, dissection of the aorta, oesophageal obstruction or perforation, disease of the spinal cord, vertebral column, ribs and skeletal musculature, subdiaphragmatic inflammation and Bornholm disease are conditions to be considered in cases of ill-defined chest pain.

Hoarseness. Acute laryngitis is the commonest cause of hoarseness. Persistent change in the voice may be due to chronic laryngitis or paresis of the left vocal cord by invasion of the recurrent laryngeal nerve by tumour.

Stridor. Loud noisy inspiration caused by obstruction of the larynx, trachea or main bronchi. In infancy acute laryngotracheobronchitis is a common cause, diphtheria is now rare. Inhalation of foreign bodies must be considered, especially in children. In adults acute inflammation and tumours are the usual causes.

Past Medical History with Special Reference to the Respiratory System. The patient should be questioned about past or present pneumonia, pleurisy and tuberculosis, and a family and contact history should be obtained. Direct questions about asthma, bronchitis and wheezing should be used. Details of childhood infections including measles and pertussis are particularly relevant where bronchiectasis is suspected. Recent onset of cough and breathlessness may follow respiratory damage at times of operations or general anesthetics.

Family History. Details to be sought include histories of tuberculosis, pneumonia and pleurisy, asthma, hay fever or allergic reactions. Family members with chronic cough, who are respiratory cripples, or who died from lung disease are often found with patients with chronic bronchitis and emphysema. A history of relatives with recurrent chest infection is common in patients with cystic fibrosis and immunological deficiencies.

Smoking History. Detailed account of the patient's total smoking history is essential. They commonly claim to be non-smokers when they have only recently stopped or reduced their smoking.

Occupational and Environmental History. Careful history of past and present occupations is essential where asthma and pulmonary fibrosis seem likely to be present. Details of family pets, travel and residence abroad should all be sought.

Chronic Obstructive Bronchitis. Commoner in workers in dusty industries such as mining, sand-blasting, woodworking, textile industries and with exposure to cadmium fumes (scrap-metal workers).

Diffuse Pulmonary Fibrosis may develop with exposure to the following industrial hazards:
1. Mining, quarrying and handling coal and silica-containing rocks.
2. Sand-blasting.
3. Stone-masonry.
4. Pottery industries.
5. Foundry work using sand.
6. Grindstone workers.
7. Boiler scalers.
8. Asbestos both in manufacture and lagging.
9. Beryllium exposure.
10. Farmers or others handling mouldy hay.
11. Mushroom workers.
12. Sugar cane handlers (bagassosis).
13. Bird handling, chicken farmers and pigeon or budgerigar keepers.

NB Exposure to asbestos, chromates and radioactive compounds is carcinogenic.

Previous Chest X-rays. Should always be sought for comparison with present films.

Chapter 2

PHYSICAL SIGNS IN CHEST DISEASE

INTRODUCTION

Examination of the respiratory system begins with observation of the patient's movements, breathing pattern and skin colour followed by systematic examination by inspection, palpation, percussion and auscultation.

INSPECTION

1. Cyanosis. This blue coloration of vascular areas of the skin and mucous membranes is present when there is about 5 g/dl of desaturated haemoglobin in the blood and its detection is affected by lighting, observer error and the patient's skin colour. With anaemia there may be insufficient haemoglobin to show cyanosis even with severe hypoxia, conversely polycythaemic patients may be cyanosed although well oxygenated.

CENTRAL CYANOSIS. Usually detectable in the mucous membranes of the mouth and conjunctivae when circulating haemoglobin is 80 per cent saturated or less (equivalent to P_aO_2 of 6·6 kPa or 50 mm Hg). Causes of central cyanosis include:

a. Ventilation–perfusion mismatching in chronic bronchitis, emphysema, asthma, bronchiectasis, pulmonary fibrosis and pulmonary emboli.

b. Hypoventilation without lung damage in drug overdose, obesity and neuromuscular disorders.

c. Right-to-left shunts in congenital heart disease (e.g. Fallot's tetralogy), intrapulmonary arteriovenous aneurysms, pneumonic consolidation and tumours.

PERIPHERAL CYANOSIS. Usually seen in the hands, feet and ears due to poor peripheral circulation caused by low cardiac output in heart failure or from cooling or other local causes of sluggish peripheral circulation.

2. Jugular Venous Pressure (JVP). This should be examined with the patient lying with the trunk at 45° to the horizontal. A raised JVP occurs in right heart failure and with severe airways obstruction the JVP may appear raised in expiration but normal emptying occurs with inspiration.

3. Shape and Symmetry of the Chest

a. BARREL-SHAPED CHEST with increase in the anteroposterior diameter is usually caused by hyperinflation and is seen with emphysema and asthma.

b. FUNNEL-SHAPED CHEST (Pectus Excavatum) is caused by depression of the lower end of the sternum and is a congenital abnormality usually of no significance. The heart may be displaced, usually to the left hemithorax.

c. PIGEON CHEST with prominence of the upper sternum is often congenital but may occur following severe persistent overinflation from asthma in childhood.

d. HARRISON'S SULCUS is a concave deformity of the lower ribs due to traction of the costal interdigitations of the diaphragm on the developing thoracic cage of children with severe airways obstruction from asthma or bronchiectasis.

e. KYPHOSCOLIOSIS, a distortion of the spine resulting in secondary deformity of the rib cage is now usually of idiopathic origin but formerly poliomyelitis was a common cause.

The breasts should always be examined for lumps. Gynaecomastia may develop in association with hypertrophic pulmonary osteo-arthropathy with bronchial neoplasms but more commonly occurs as a side effect of drugs such as spironolactone or digoxin.

4. Chest Movement. Respiratory rate, rhythm and depth should be observed. Unilateral causes of reduced chest wall movement include pulmonary collapse, pneumonic consolidation, pleural effusion, pneumothorax and localized pulmonary fibrosis. Bilateral loss of chest wall movement occurs in chronic bronchitis, emphysema and diffuse pulmonary fibrosis and more rarely with neuromuscular disorders and ankylosing spondylitis.

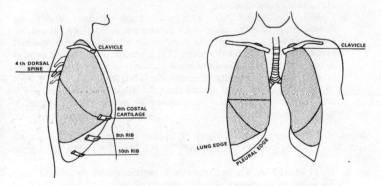

Fig. 1. Surface anatomy of the lungs. Anterior view and lateral view of the right lung at functional residual capacity.

5. Surface Anatomy of the Thorax (*Fig.* 1). The following landmarks should be recognized:

The *sternal angle* anteriorly at the level of the 2nd rib is opposite the tracheal bifurcation.

The oblique fissure may be traced around from the 2nd thoracic spine posteriorly to the 6th costochondral junction anteriorly.

The right horizontal fissure follows the 4th intercostal space anteriorly to the midaxillary line.

6. Finger Clubbing. The earliest sign is loss of the angle between the nail and the dorsum of the terminal phalanx with shiny, sponginess of the skin at the nail bed. Later curvature of the nail increases until the tip of the finger becomes swollen with a drumstick appearance.

Causes of finger clubbing:

a. RESPIRATORY. Bronchial carcinoma, more rarely mesothelioma of the pleura, mediastinal tumours including thymoma and Hodgkin's disease. Formerly it was common with intrapulmonary sepsis especially bronchiectasis, but also tuberculosis, lung abscess and empyema. Clubbing is common with some fibrosing lung diseases such as cryptogenic fibrosing alveolitis and asbestosis, but is rare with sarcoidosis.

b. CARDIOVASCULAR. Intracardiac right-to-left shunts in cyanotic congenital heart lesions, pulmonary arteriovenous aneurysms, bacterial endocarditis and aortic aneurysm.

c. GASTROINTESTINAL DISEASE. Chronic diarrhoea, especially ulcerative colitis and less often Crohn's disease and coeliac disease. Chronic hepatic fibrosis from biliary cirrhosis or portal cirrhosis may cause finger clubbing.

d. FAMILIAL CLUBBING. This may occur without underlying disease. Hypertrophic pulmonary osteoarthropathy (HPA) is usually accompanied by clubbing and is especially associated with bronchial carcinoma and pleural fibromas. It is characterized by warm painful swelling of the wrists and ankles. A minority of cases show gynaecomastia. On radiography an irregular periosteal reaction is best recognized at the distal end of the tibia-fibula or radius-ulna. HPA associated with pulmonary neoplasms may regress when the primary tumour is excised.

Signs of Respiratory Failure. Signs of hypercapnia and hypoxia are non-specific and these conditions may not be recognized on clinical examination.

a. HYPERCAPNIA. Carbon dioxide retention causes peripheral vasodilatation with engorged veins and a full bounding pulse. Cerebral effects include drowsiness, intellectual impairment and disorientation progressing to coma. Headache from cerebral vasodilatation is common and rarely there may be papilloedema. A jerky flapping tremor of the hands is common.

b. HYPOXIA. This also may cause intellectual impairment, behavioural disturbance and irritability leading to drowsiness and coma. Cardiac dysrhythmias are common with hypoxia.

PALPATION

1. Position of Mediastinum. The trachea in the suprasternal notch should be felt with the fingers. *Deviation* of the trachea to the opposite side occurs with thyroid swellings, cervical and superior mediastinal lymph-gland enlargement. Traction of the trachea to the affected side occurs with fibrosis of the lung apices and upper lobe collapse.

DISPLACEMENT OF THE LOWER MEDIASTINUM, recognized by shift of the apex beat, may be caused by a pleural effusion or pneumothorax leading to displacement to the opposite side. Displacement to the affected side may result from pulmonary fibrosis or collapse of a lung.

2. Chest Expansion. Estimated by placing the hands symmetrically on each side of the chest or more accurately with a tape measure in the midthoracic region. Reduced expansion is common with chronic airways obstruction or pulmonary fibrosis.

3. Tactile Vocal Fremitus. Vocal vibrations may be felt by placing the ulnar border of the hand on the chest wall as the patient repeats 'ninety-nine'. Vocal fremitus (vibrations) will be reduced over a pneumothorax or pleural effusion and increased by consolidation of the lung and pulmonary fibrosis.

PERCUSSION

Middle finger of the left hand is placed along the line of a rib and is struck by the middle finger of the right hand. Dullness to percussion occurs over a pleural effusion, pulmonary collapse, localized pulmonary or pleural fibrosis and pneumonic consolidation. Resonance is increased over a pneumothorax and overinflated lungs in asthma or emphysema. Loss of the cardiac and liver areas of dullness is common with overinflation of the chest.

AUSCULTATION

To elicit breath sounds and adventitious sounds.

Breath Sounds

Normal breath sounds are rustling and high pitched, inspiratory sounds are louder and shorter than expiratory sounds.

Bronchial breathing is recognized as low pitched sounds with a blowing quality. It may be simulated by listening over the trachea. Bronchial breathing may be heard over pneumonic consolidation, localized pulmonary fibrosis and above large pleural effusions.

Amphoric breathing is heard over large cavities.

Reduced breath sounds occur with pulmonary collapse, pneumonia, emphysema, pleural fibrosis or effusion and pneumothorax or obstruction of a large bronchus by a neoplasm or foreign body.

Adventitious Sounds. Wheezes (rhonchi), crackles (crepitations or râles) and pleural rubs.

1. WHEEZES OR RHONCHI are continuous sounds caused by air flow through bronchi on the point of collapse. May be high or low pitched and audible in inspiration and/or expiration. Wheezes occur with all forms of generalized airways obstruction including asthma, chronic bronchitis and bronchiectasis. Localized wheeze may result from partial obstruction of a bronchus by mucus, tumour or a foreign body. Pitch and loudness of wheezes do not indicate the size of bronchus affected but with severe airflow obstruction wheezes will become quieter.

2. CRACKLES OR CREPITATIONS are generated by explosive re-opening of smaller airways, bronchi or bronchioles, which are closed due to deflation of the lung resulting from the presence of space-occupying material such as oedema fluid, inflammatory exudates or fibrous tissue. Are usually best heard in dependent parts of lungs where effects of gravity cause greatest deflation. As the lung inflates on inspiration, equalization of pressure occurs across the closed segment of an airway between the open proximal portion and the trapped air in the alveoli. Sudden opening of the closed portion of the airway occurs giving the crackle or crepitation. Timing or intensity of the crackles is dependent on the size of airway affected. In early disease when the space-occupying material first accumulates only the smaller airways are affected and fine crackles are heard near to full inflation i.e. at late inspiration. With more extensive oedema or fibrosis and especially where the bronchial walls are abnormal (e.g. bronchiectasis) louder crackles may be heard earlier in inspiration.

3. PLEURAL RUB. Pleural inflammation with pulmonary infarction, pneumonia or neoplastic infiltration may be accompanied by a creaking sound present on inspiration and expiration.

4. AN INTRATHORACIC SPLASH. Due to presence of air and fluid in a hydropneumothorax or within a hiatus hernia; may occasionally be heard by shaking the patient.

SIGNS OF LOCAL DISEASE IN THE CHEST

1. Consolidation. Movement of the affected side is reduced, the percussion note is dull, vocal fremitus is reduced and bronchial breathing is audible. There may be pan-inspiratory or late inspiratory crackles depending on the extent of lung involved. Vocal resonance may have a bleating quality ('aegophony').

Whispering pectoriloquy may be present i.e. whispered speech is amplified on auscultation with the stethoscope.

2. Collapse. With loss of lung volume caused by collapse there is impaired movement of the affected side and with upper lobe collapse the trachea may be deviated to that side. With extensive lower lobe collapse the apex beat may be displaced to the affected side. Breath sounds are diminished or absent over a collapsed lobe or lung.

3. Pleural Effusion. Movement of the affected side is reduced, the apex beat may be displaced to the opposite side and very rarely with a very large effusion the trachea may be similarly affected. The percussion note is dull, vocal fremitus and breath sounds are absent.

4. Pneumothorax without Tension. The percussion note is normal. Breath sounds are diminished or absent. The apex beat may be displaced and the area of cardiac dullness may be lost.

5. Tension Pneumothorax. This causes displacement of the trachea and apex beat away from the affected side. There is severe reduction of movement. Cyanosis and respiratory distress with pulsus paradoxus and hypotension will develop rapidly.

Chapter 3

THE CHEST X-RAY

Plain X-rays of the chest are probably the single most useful investigation in chest disease.

In order that abnormalities are not overlooked it is essential to use an orderly sequence of examination looking first for normal anatomical structures and then for abnormal shadows. Begin by checking the name and date on the radiograph and whether the film has been taken in the standard postero-anterior (PA) position, or as a portable anteroposterior (AP) view as this will magnify the heart and major vessel shadows. The position of the patient at X-ray can be assessed by looking at the medial ends of each clavicle which should be evenly disposed on either side of the vertebral bodies. A useful system is to begin with soft tissues and thoracic cage, followed by diaphragm, heart shadow, trachea, hilar shadows, lung vessels, horizontal fissure, lung density or blackness. Each aspect will be dealt with in turn, normal structures followed by abnormal features.

SOFT TISSUES

In women the breast and nipple shadows should be noted and in men those of the pectoralis muscles. Obesity may show as horizontal lines caused by folds of flesh.

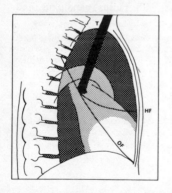 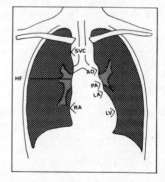

Fig. 2. The chest X-ray. Postero-anterior and right lateral views. SVC, superior vena cava; Ao, aortic knuckle; PA, pulmonary artery; LA, left atrium; LV, left ventricle; RA, right atrium; HF, horizontal fissures; OF, oblique fissure; T, trachea.

THORACIC CAGE

Symmetry of the skeleton should be looked for, the intercostal spaces should be equal in width on the two sides. Abnormalities to be noted include unilateral crowding of the ribs in kyphoscoliosis or due to loss of lung volume through collapse or resection of lung tissue. The rib margins should be examined for irregularities resulting from trauma, fractures, infection or erosion by tumour. Notching of the posterior portion of the ribs and scapulae occurs with coarctation of the aorta.

DIAPHRAGM

The right dome should be 1–2 cm higher than the left and opposite the anterior end of the 5th or 6th ribs. It should have a clear outline throughout, but may be obscured by large breast shadows. Elevation of the diaphragm may occur with increase in intra-abdominal pressure due to ascites, obesity and pregnancy. Unilateral elevation of the diaphragm may be caused by excess gas in the stomach, subphrenic abscess, collapse of the middle or lower lobe on the affected side, phrenic nerve paralysis, from trauma, malignant disease, lymph node enlargement or spinal curvature.

HEART SHADOW

The transverse diameter of the heart should be less than half the maximum diameter of the thoracic cage and in normal subjects ranges from 11·5 to 15·5 cm. The shape of the heart should be noticed and any prominence of the aortic knuckle and the main ventricular mass should be observed. One-third of the heart lies to the right of the spine in normal subjects. Displacement of the heart shadow to one side may occur with spinal deformities such as kyphoscoliosis and pectus excavatum, as a result of loss of lung volume from collapse of the lung or the presence of a pneumothorax or pleural effusion.

TRACHEA

This should be visible as a vertical translucent band overlying the spinous processes of the upper thoracic vertebrae. Collapse or fibrosis of an upper lobe and upper mediastinal tumours will cause deviation of the trachea.

HILAR SHADOWS

These are composed of the pulmonary vessels. The left hilum shadow is about 1–2 cm higher than the right. Bilateral enlargement of the hilar vessel shadows occurs in pulmonary hypertension. Other causes include sarcoidosis, Hodgkin's disease, lymphosarcoma, leukaemia, tuberculosis,

Fig. 3. See opposite.

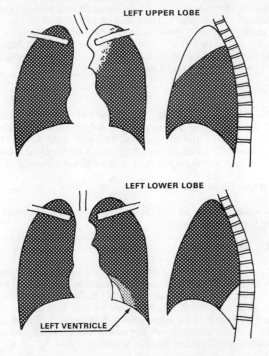

Fig. 3. Diagrams of the radiographic changes produced by lobar collapse.

malignant metastases and aortic aneurysm. Unilateral enlargement of the hilar shadow occurs with carcinoma of the bronchus and both tuberculosis and sarcoidosis may occasionally present as unilateral enlargement.

LUNG VESSELS

These should be traced from the periphery to the hila. In areas where the lung is partially collapsed the vessels may be crowded together and the translucency of the lung reduced. In areas of hyperinflation the vessels will be further apart and the lung will appear more radiolucent. In emphysema where there is destruction of the alveolar tissues the vascular pattern will be attenuated, especially towards the periphery of the lung fields. In congestion of the pulmonary circulation as in left heart failure or with mitral stenosis the vascular pattern will be accentuated and in pulmonary oedema make fan-shaped shadows, spreading out from the hilar region. In addition to this, hair-like shadows at the margins of the lungs approximately at right angles to the lateral chest wall (Kerley B lines) are caused by fluid accentuating the interlobular connective-tissue septa.

LOBES AND FISSURES

In the PA film in 50–60 per cent of patients the horizontal fissure is visible at the level of the anterior end of the 4th rib and the 6th rib in the axilla. On a lateral film the oblique fissure runs from the 4th or 5th thoracic vertebra downwards through the hilum to the anterior costophrenic angle. Collapse of a lobe will draw the fissures towards the collapsed area (*Fig. 3*).

ABNORMAL SHADOWS

Any abnormal shadow should be analysed for its anatomical site, size, shape and nature of its margins.

CONSOLIDATED LOBES

Consolidation from any cause gives a uniform opacity, the dimensions of which remain approximately normal and if the bronchi are patent they may be visible as an air bronchogram. Collapse of lung is identified by reduction in size of the affected segment or lobe with altered position of the fissures. Collapse of an upper lobe will cause deviation of the tracheal translucency to the affected side and collapse of a lower lobe may displace the mediastinal structures to the side affected.

SOFT-TISSUE MASSES

Lung tumours may appear as expansions of the hilar shadow or as peripheral shadows. Round shadows near the periphery may be any one of a number of different lesions, the nature of which cannot be decided purely on X-ray appearances.

INFLAMMATORY LESIONS

A wide variety of appearances may result from different lung pathologies.

PLEURAL EFFUSIONS

Present a uniform opacity obliterating other soft-tissue shadows, extending upwards from the costophrenic angles. There will be a concave upper margin for optical reasons unless air is also present in the pleural space when a horizontal upper border to the shadow will be present.

PNEUMOTHORAX

With a small pneumothorax a hairline shadow may be just visible along the lung edge. This may be more easily seen by taking films in full expiration when increased pressure in the air in the pneumothorax increases its size and the greater radiodensity of the compressed lung tissue more easily contrasts with the radiolucent pneumothorax. Emphysematous bullae may be seen as hairline curvilinear shadows. Thicker linear shadows, especially with fluid levels, suggest cavitating lesions such as a lung abscess or tumour.

SPECIAL TECHNIQUES

1. Tomography. Useful for demonstrating pulmonary cavities, the lumen of the trachea and major bronchi, any stenosis of these airways and the presence of intraluminal masses. AP tomograms are particularly useful for defining lesions in the upper lobes while lateral tomograms are best for middle and lower lobe shadows. For lesions of the hila both AP and lateral tomography may be necessary.

2. Bronchography. By the use of radio-opaque iodized oil a detailed silhouette of the bronchial anatomy can be produced. This is valuable for demonstrating the presence or extent of bronchiectasis, small endo-bronchial lesions and more peripheral sites of airways obstruction. It is a particularly useful technique for the investigation of haemoptysis.

3. Fluoroscopy. This is valuable for assessing diaphragmatic movement. It must be done with the patient prone or supine because in the erect position movement of the abdominal wall may be transmitted through the abdominal contents to the diaphragm giving spurious movement in the presence of diaphragmatic paresis.

4. Isotope Techniques. The distribution of the pulmonary arterial circulation can be estimated by scanning over the lung fields after intravenous injection of macroaggregates of human albumin labelled with [131]Iodine or [99m]Technetium. The distribution of ventilation can be assessed by scanning after inhalation of [133]Xenon, [89m]Krypton or other suitable insoluble radioactive gases. Interpretation of the results is beyond the scope of this book.

Chapter 4

CARDIOVASCULAR ASPECTS OF LUNG DISEASE

The following clinical abnormalities of the cardiovascular system may commonly be encountered in lung disease.

Pulse
1. TACHYCARDIA may indicate hypoxaemia in asthma, exacerbations of chronic bronchitis and other causes of respiratory failure.
2. WIDE PULSE PRESSURE with dilatation of the peripheral and retinal veins and rarely papilloedema occurs with hypercapnia.
3. PULSUS PARADOXUS is a common physical sign in patients with severe airways obstruction. It is the cyclical variation of systolic blood pressure with inspiration and expiration. Its genesis is complex but is related to the effects of wide swings in intrathoracic pressure on left ventricular volume. It may be detectable by palpation when the degree of paradox i.e. the difference between systolic blood pressure in inspiration and expiration, is greater than 20 mm Hg. It may be quantified with the sphygmomanometer. The cuff is blown up until all sounds are obliterated. As the pressure in the cuff is lowered the systolic sound will first be heard only in expiration, this pressure should be noted. As the cuff pressure is lowered further the systolic sound will be heard in inspiration also, the difference between this reading and the previous pressure is the degree of pulsus paradoxus. In acute asthma it has been shown to be closely related to the severity of airways obstruction and the degree of carbon dioxide retention.
4. DIFFERENCE IN PULSE VOLUME. Rarely the pulse volume in the two arms may be different as a result of an apical carcinoma of the lung affecting the brachial plexus.

Jugular Venous Pressure (JVP). This should be assessed with the patient reclining at an angle of 45°.
1. RIGHT HEART FAILURE secondary to chronic lung disease is the commonest cause of a raised JVP in lung disease. There may be associated oedema of the dependent parts, liver engorgement and signs of right ventricular hypertrophy and a pansystolic murmur of tricuspid regurgitation.
2. FLUCTUATIONS WITH RESPIRATION. A raised JVP in expiration with normal pressure on inspiration is a common feature of severe airways obstruction. Venous return is obstructed by the increase in intrathoracic pressure which occurs with expiration.
3. SUPERIOR VENA CAVAL OBSTRUCTION. This will cause persistent engorgement of the neck veins and associated plethora and

cyanosis of the face, neck and arms. It is usually caused by bronchial carcinoma — rarer causes are lymphomas and fibrosing mediastinitis.

Examination of the Heart

1. ABSENCE OF THE APEX BEAT AND LOSS OF CARDIAC DULLNESS. These are probably the commonest abnormal cardiac signs of lung diseases and are caused by overinflation of the lungs in bronchitis, emphysema and asthma, and with a pneumothorax.

2. PARASTERNAL HEAVE. May develop with right ventricular hypertrophy secondary to severe chronic lung disease i.e. cor pulmonale.

3. HEART SOUNDS

   a. *Diminution in Intensity* of the heart sounds because of overinflation is a common abnormal finding in chronic respiratory diseases. Rarely the second heart sound may be reduced in intensity in pulmonary stenosis.

   b. *Increased Intensity*. The first heart sound and the pulmonary component of the second sound may be increased in intensity in pulmonary hypertension. Splitting of the second sound may be accentuated or fixed in inspiration and expiration with pulmonary hypertension.

   c. *Third and Fourth Heart Sounds*. The third heart sound due to ventricular filling and fourth heart sound in late diastole due to atrial contraction and rapid ventricular filling may be accentuated in the presence of pulmonary hypertension and right ventricular failure.

4. CARDIAC MURMURS. Arising from the right heart are much less common than left heart murmurs.

   a. *Pansystolic Blowing Murmur*. Audible at the base in tricuspid regurgitation may develop secondary to right ventricular hypertrophy. It is accompanied by giant 'V' waves in the JVP and sometimes pulsatile enlargement of the liver.

   b. *Midsystolic Ejection Murmur*. This may be audible with pulmonary valve stenosis.

   c. *Early Diastolic Murmur*. A high pitched murmur may be heard with pulmonary regurgitation but this is rare.

PULMONARY OEDEMA

Causes to be considered include:

1. *Left Heart Diseases*. These are the commonest causes and include left ventricular failure from systemic hypertension, ischaemic heart disease or valve defect secondary to left atrial hypertension as in mitral stenosis.

2. *Fluid and Electrolyte Overload*. In renal failure, liver failure. Iatrogenic causes are common and include overtransfusion of blood or intravenous fluids.

3. *Noxious Gases.* These may damage pulmonary capillaries and alveolar lining cells. Examples are chlorine and oxides of nitrogen.

4. *Neurogenic Mechanisms.* Including head injury, intracerebral tumour or cerebrovascular haemorrhage may rarely cause pulmonary oedema.

5. *Re-expansion Pulmonary Oedema.* This may develop following too rapid removal of air or fluid from the pleural space.

6. *Drugs.* Heroin and some other drugs may occasionally cause pulmonary oedema.

Pathophysiology. Initially any increase in intrapulmonary fluid will be dealt with by lymphatic drainage but if this is reduced or ineffective further increase in filtration from the pulmonary vessels through the interstitial space of the lungs leads to an oedema cuff around the airways and blood vessels. Subsequently alveolar oedema will occur, lifting the surfactant layer away from the alveolar walls. Under the influence of gravity this fluid accumulation will be greatest in the dependent parts of the lungs.

Respiratory Effects

1. AIRWAY NARROWING. Affects the non-cartilage-containing airways, first causing crackles but with severe oedema, larger airways may be affected and wheezes may be audible.

2. LOSS OF COMPLIANCE. Stiffening of the lungs by engorgement of the interstitial tissues leads to reduced compliance or distensibility.

3. REDISTRIBUTION OF VENTILATION. Away from the dependent zones of the lungs to the more compliant upper zones. This is accompanied by changes in perfusion resulting from local hypoxic and reflex contriction of arterioles.

4. HYPERPNOEA. Develops probably due to stimulation of the irritant juxtacapillary or J-receptors in the lungs.

Clinical Features

1. BREATHLESSNESS. If pulmonary oedema is mild, breathlessness may only be noticeable on exercise.

2. PAROXYSMAL NOCTURNAL DYSPNOEA

3. ORTHOPNOEA. This must be differentiated from other cause of nocturnal breathlessness, such as severe airways obstruction.

4. COUGH. This is often unproductive, but with severe pulmonary oedema it is accompanied by breathlessness, cyanosis and frothy sputum.

5. CHEYNE–STOKES RESPIRATION. This cyclical breathing with apnoeic periods is usually a sign of advanced heart disease. The clinical signs are non-specific and in very early pulmonary oedema without radiographic change fine late inspiratory crackles may be audible at the lung bases. As the severity of the oedema increases

crackles become earlier in inspiration because the increasing fluid leads to the closure of larger more proximal airways.

Chest X-Ray

1. Mildest degrees of oedema will show as upper lobe venous engorgement and relative narrowing of lower lobe veins.
2. More marked oedema gives perihilar 'fluffy' shadows.
3. With well established oedema, horizontal Kerley B lines are present and are best seen at the outer margins of the lungs in the lower zones.
4. PLEURAL EFFUSION. With gross pulmonary oedema pleural effusions develop. These are usually bilateral but if unilateral, the left side is most often affected. They are caused by accentuation of the interlobular connective-tissue septa by fluid accumulation.
5. HEART SIZE. Cardiac enlargement may develop due to dilatation of the left ventricle.

Functional Disturbances. Pulmonary oedema presents with a restrictive ventilatory defect but gas transfer may be increased due to the engorgement of pulmonary vessels. More severe degrees of oedema may result in airways obstruction with loss of static lung volumes. Hyperventilation caused by loss of compliance and increased J-receptor nervous impulses usually results in hypocapnia with associated hypoxaemia. With more severe pulmonary oedema carbon dioxide retention may develop and a metabolic acidosis may also develop from tissue hypoxia.

Treatment

1. Of the primary disturbance, wherever possible.
2. Oxygen in high concentrations (35–50 per cent).
3. I.v. diuretics e.g. frusemide.
4. In very severe pulmonary oedema unresponsive to frusemide venesection either by the use of limb cuffs or by blood letting may still be necessary.
5. Morphine or heroin may have specific effects.
6. Aminophylline by i.v. injection may help ease breathlessness by relieving airways obstruction.
7. Intermittent partial-pressure ventilation may be necessary for the most severe degrees of pulmonary oedema.

Chapter 5

THE FORM AND FUNCTION OF THE LUNGS

Respiration is the means by which all cells in the body live consuming oxygen and producing carbon dioxide. These gases are transported to and from the cells through the blood and tissue fluids and are exchanged with atmospheric air at the lungs. The main design feature of the lungs is that air is brought into contact with venous blood at the alveoli over as large a surface area as possible with the minimum of intervening tissue. Gas exchange is the primary function of the lungs but they also participate in a number of other metabolic processes.

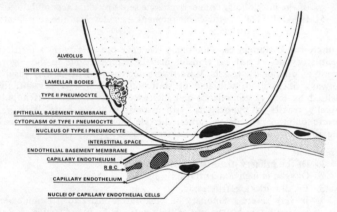

ALVEOLUS

INTER CELLULAR BRIDGE

LAMELLAR BODIES

TYPE II PNEUMOCYTE

EPITHELIAL BASEMENT MEMBRANE
CYTOPLASM OF TYPE I PNEUMOCYTE
NUCLEUS OF TYPE I PNEUMOCYTE

INTERSTITIAL SPACE
ENDOTHELIAL BASEMENT MEMBRANE
CAPILLARY ENDOTHELIUM
R B C

CAPILLARY ENDOTHELIUM

NUCLEI OF CAPILLARY ENDOTHELIAL CELLS

Fig. 4. The structure of the alveolar wall drawn from an electron-photomicrograph. Note that the blood—gas barrier consists of the epithelium of a type 1 pneumonocyte with its basement membrane, interstitial tissue and the capillary endothelium and its basement membrane.

THE ALVEOLUS

There are about 300 million alveoli in the adult lung providing a surface area for gas exchange of about 100 m². The blood—gas barrier is about 1 μm thick, and is composed of a respiratory epithelial cell and a capillary endothelial cell each with a basement membrane and a small interstitial space between them (*Fig.* 4). The interstitial space contains elastic and collagen fibres as well as connective-tissue cells. The cells of the alveolar epithelium are of two kinds, the Type 1 pneumonocyte which is a large flat cell and the cytoplasm of which forms most of the epithelial wall of the alveolus, covering a surface area about 20 times as large as that of the Type 2 pneumonocyte which is a more compact cell with lamellated osmiophilic inclusion bodies which are probably the origin of surfactant, a fluid of low surface tension which lines the alveoli and airways helping to maintain their patency. Judged by the number of nuclei present there are 50 per cent more Type 2 than Type 1 pneumonocytes within each alveolus.

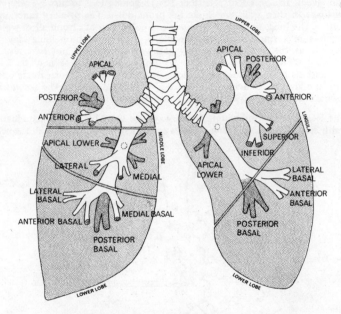

Fig. 5. The tracheobronchial tree and lung segments.

THE AIRWAYS

Inspired air passes through the nose and pharynx where it is warmed and humidified by a richly vascular mucosa and then passes through the larynx and trachea before entering the complex system of branching airways. The trachea divides into right and left main bronchi which then give off lobar and segmental bronchi (*Fig.* 5). Thereafter there are two main types of intrasegmental pathways, *axial* airways which run the longest possible course, passing directly from the hilum to the distal pleura, and *lateral* airways supplying regions between the hilum and the distal pleural surface. Bronchi are defined as tubes containing cartilage within their walls. There are about five generations of 'large' bronchi in which the rings or plates of cartilage are sufficiently large that any cross-sectional cut will include some cartilage. Then follow between 5 and 10 further generations of 'small' bronchi where cartilage is reduced to small plates so that some cross-sectional cuts may show no cartilage. Between the last bronchus and the alveoli is a series of a further 10—15 generations of airways without cartilage in their walls which are the bronchioles. The primary functional unit of the lung, the *acinus* (*Fig.* 6), is a collection of alveoli all of which stem from a single terminal bronchiole. A terminal bronchiole may be defined as the last airway in any pathway which does not have alveoli opening directly from its walls. Within an acinus there may be 3—8 generations of respiratory bronchioles and from these alveolar ducts open into the alveoli. An acinus is about 0·5—1 cm in diameter. The *secondary lobule* is composed of 3—5 terminal bronchioles with their acini.

The Respiratory Epithelium. The airways are lined by a columnar ciliated epithelium which in the large airways appears stratified because all the cells

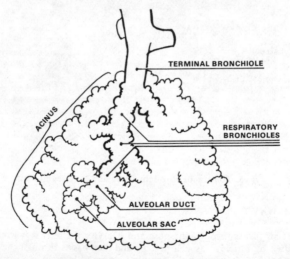

Fig. 6. The acinus or primary lobule. The acinus comprises the respiratory bronchioles and alveoli supplied by one terminal bronchiole. Each acinus contains up to three generations of respiratory bronchioles from which the alveolar ducts lead to the alveolar sacs from which the alveoli open.

reach the basement membrane, but the basal cell does not reach the surface. In the smaller airways, all the cells reach the surface. The types of cells so far identified include *goblet* cells which secrete an acid glycoprotein which, mixed with a transudate produced by the non-ciliated cells, lines the airways and provides a coat covering the cilia. *Ciliated cells* form a continuous system from the junction of the respiratory bronchioles and alveolar ducts right up to the nares. The *brush cell,* of which there are relatively few, resembles similar cells with microvilli found in the gut and may control fluid balance in the lung by absorption or secretion. The *basal cell* may not have a specific function but is probably capable of differentiating to replace goblet cells or ciliated cells. *Kulchitsky cells* are believed to receive a neural innervation and may be a source of kinins and other mediators of lung metabolism. *Clara cells* are plentiful and with their abundant cytoplasm are probably secretory cells. It has been suggested that they are the source of surfactant but it seems more likely that this is secreted by the Type 2 pneumonocytes within the alveoli.

The Submucosal Glands. The bronchial submucosal glands are both serous and mucous in type. Several forms of acid glycoprotein, sialic acid and sulphate are produced in their secretions.

DEVELOPMENT OF THE LUNGS

The trachea develops from the foregut during the 4th week of intra-uterine life and the branching pattern of airways develops rapidly so that the lobar and segmental airways are present by the 5th week, and the adult pattern of airways is complete by the 16th week in utero. The cartilage and glandular structures are all present by the 28th week in utero. At birth there are about 20 million primitive alveoli present and a phase of rapid multiplication occurs until the age of 3 years, thereafter multiplication slows but the alveoli increase in size to match the growth of the thorax so that the adult complement of 300 million alveoli is present by 8 years of age. Development of the pulmonary circulation matches that of the airways. The pre-acinar vessels are all present by 16 weeks in utero and the acinar vessels develop as the alveoli multiply. Muscularization of the acinar vessels does not become fully developed until early adult life.

THE GROSS ANATOMY OF THE LUNG

The lungs are divided into three lobes on the right and two on the left (*see Fig.* 5). Each lobe is completely invested in parietal pleura which is reflected from one lobe to another at the hilum. The lobes are subdivided into bronchopulmonary segments by fibrous tissue septa extending inwards from the pleural surface. The lobar bronchus divides within each lobe into segmental bronchi from which there are then successive subdivisions on to bronchioles. The right main bronchus is shorter than the left and more vertically in line with the trachea, as a result inhaled material is more likely to enter the right lung. The tracheal wall contains the U-shaped cartilaginous rings supporting the anterior and lateral walls. The posterior wall is composed of longitudinal and transverse elastic fibres and during coughing and other causes of increased intrathoracic pressure it is drawn forward, reducing the lumen of the trachea to a crescentic slit. As a result, airflow of high linear velocity is produced and this aids in the clearance of secretions and inhaled particles.

THE PULMONARY CIRCULATION

There are two complete vascular systems in the lungs. The pulmonary arteries arise from the right ventricle and supply the capillary bed within the alveolar walls, and the bronchial arteries arise from the aorta to supply the capillary bed in the walls of the bronchi and bronchioles. Each airway is accompanied by branches of the pulmonary artery and the pulmonary vein which are contained within a loose connective tissue sheath as a *bronchovascular bundle*. Within the bronchial walls there are branches of the bronchial artery. The pulmonary veins drain to the left atrium receiving blood from the whole of the intrapulmonary capillary bed, both from the alveoli and the airways. The bronchial veins receive blood from the hilum, the large airways, pleura and lymph nodes and drain to the azygos system. There are precapillary anastomoses between the pulmonary and bronchial arteries. The main and segmental branches of the pulmonary artery have elastic walls, this changes to a muscular coat in the arteries within a segment of the lung. The smaller arteries show a less marked muscular coat and the precapillary arteries are non-muscular.

THE LYMPHATICS

There are no lymphatics within the alveolar walls but they are plentiful in the connective tissue of the pleura, the interlobular septa and the walls of the airways, arteries and veins. Some of the lymphatic channels follow the airways while others take more circuitous routes so that drainage from different units may be mixed together. There are small collections of lymphocytes within the lobules of the lung and larger and more numerous collections at the junction of segments and lobes. Lymphatic drainage is from the periphery towards the hilum.

THE NERVES

The pulmonary vessels and connective tissue of the lungs are richly supplied from both parasympathetic and sympathetic systems but as yet identifiable nerve endings have not been found in the alveolar walls in man. Juxta-capillary or J-receptors have been found at the centre of acini in certain species. These are thought to initiate rapid shallow breathing but they have not yet been identified in the human lung. Sensory nerve endings have been identified in human tracheal epithelium and in other species both sensory and motor terminals have been found within the epithelium of other airways.

THE CONNECTIVE TISSUE

The lungs are rich in connective tissue, that surrounding the bronchial blood vessels in the bronchovascular bundles is in continuity with the connective tissue within the alveolar walls. In some parts of the lungs there are connective-tissue septa arising from the pleura and penetrating the lung substance at approximately right angles to the pleural surface. These septa are incomplete in man but are most marked at the margins and sharp edges of the lungs such as the anterior edges of the upper lobes and lingula, the costodiaphragmatic rim and the posteromedial margins of the lungs. These septa are the structures seen as Kerley B lines on chest X-rays when they are accentuated by the presence of pulmonary oedema, cellular infiltration or fibrosis.

COLLATERAL VENTILATION

Because the connective-tissue septa in man are incomplete, collateral ventilation or airdrift from one alveolus to another and one lobule to another is possible. For this reason the lung distal to occluded airways may be prevented from collapse. Several different interalveolar or intersegmental connections have been recognized.

Canals of Lambert. These connect respiratory bronchioles, terminal bronchioles and possibly other larger airways to alveoli and alveolar ducts supplied by other airways. They are certainly present within the infant lung but their numbers and site in adult lung is uncertain.

Accessory Bronchiolo-alveolar Communications. These are lined by a continuous layer of epithelium and are small channels passing between terminal and preterminal bronchioli and alveolar ducts of adjacent alveoli. Present in dog lungs but it is not yet certain whether they exist in man.

Pores of Kohn. All alveoli are in direct continuity with their neighbours through these gaps in the alveolar walls.

Double Diffusion. Because diffusion across the blood—gas barrier is very rapid it is possible that gas tensions may equalize in adjacent alveoli by simple gaseous diffusion.

Collateral ventilation is slower and less effective in children because these interalveolar connections are not fully developed until several years after birth.

BREATHING

Breathing is an involuntary act which may be modified by voluntary effort. In the intact subject the lungs are always somewhat distended and positive elastic forces are present which would tend to collapse the lungs if they were not held against the rib cage by surface tension forces between the parietal and visceral layers of pleura. If the thoracic cage is opened at operation the lungs will deflate due to this stored elastic tension and occupy a smaller volume than that which they do in the intact chest. Under resting conditions, inspiration is brought about by contraction and descent of the diaphragm and upward and outward movement of the rib cage through contraction of the external intercostal muscles. In quiet expiration the lungs and rib cage return to their resting position through release of the elastic tension stored in the stretched lungs and by graded relaxation of the inspiratory muscles. In rapid or deep breathing and in association with diseases with airways obstruction or increased stiffness of the lungs inspiration is aided by active contraction of the sternomastoid and strap muscles of the neck and expiration is assisted by active contraction of the muscles of the abdominal wall.

THE ALVEOLI AND GAS-EXCHANGING SURFACE

The alveoli in all parts of the lung are probably of the same potential size but the balance of forces affecting alveolar size is such that alveoli in the upper part are usually more distended than those at the bases. In the upper zones pleural pressure is negative with respect to atmosphere and is counterbalanced by the elastic recoil pressure of the lungs. In the lower zones, pleural pressure is greater because of the effects of the weight of the overlying lung and this tends, therefore, to reduce alveolar and airway size. However, the change in volume of the alveoli with respiration is greater in the lower zones than in the upper zones so that under resting conditions most ventilation occurs in the dependent parts of the lungs.

In inspiration, air enters the lungs through the single trachea and the majority of resistance to airflow in normal individuals resides in the large central airways of the first four or five generations of bronchi. At this level, airflow is turbulent. Within the next few generations of airways there is a progressive rapid increase in the total cross-sectional area of the bronchial tree resulting in a marked fall in resistance to flow and the airflow changes to laminar (*Fig.* 7). In inspiration and expiration air moves by bulk flow up and down the airways as far as the region of the respiratory bronchioles but beyond this point gas exchange to the alveoli and thence to the blood in the pulmonary capillaries occurs by molecular diffusion. During inspiration the elastic traction or recoil of the lungs helps to maintain airway calibre. During expiration elastic traction diminishes and the increase in intrathoracic pressure tends to narrow the airways. Thus, airways resistance is lower in inspiration than expiration. A number of factors will influence airway calibre including the distensibility of individual airways, their inherent stability which is dependent upon the presence of surfactant and the clearance of secretions, the thickness of the respiratory epithelium, the quantity of glandular tissue within the airway wall, and the state of contraction of the smooth muscle within the airway wall.

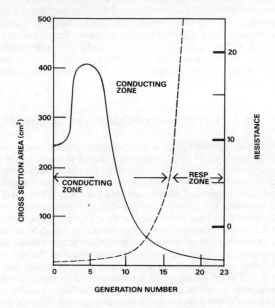

RESISTANCE cm H$_2$O/L/SEC $\times$ 10^3

Fig. 7. This shows the relationship between the total cross-sectional area of the tracheobronchial tree and the resistance to gas flow. Note that after about the tenth generation of airways, there is a sharp fall in the resistance to gas flow because of a marked increase in the cross-sectional area of the airways.

DISTRIBUTION OF VENTILATION

In the normal lung, although all the alveoli are probably of the same potential size and structure they vary in their volume in different regions of the lungs because of the influence of gravity and intrathoracic pressure. The lungs are suspended within the chest not from the hilum but as a result of adhesion between the visceral and parietal layers of pleura. In upright animals like man the alveoli in the upper lobes are more distended than those in the lower lobes at all phases of respiration except full inflation (total lung capacity, TLC). Similarly, the airways, especially the smaller bronchi and bronchioles, will be more dilated in the upper zones than in the lower zones. Of the air drawn into the lungs about 150 ml fills the airways down to the level of the terminal bronchioles, this is referred to as the *anatomical dead space*. Even in the normal lungs, not all of the air reaching the alveoli is effectively used in gas exchange because there are some alveoli which, although well ventilated, are poorly perfused. The volume of air occupying such alveoli is referred to as the *physiological dead space*. In a variety of diseases the volume of this physiological dead space is increased.

DISTRIBUTION OF PERFUSION (PULMONARY HAEMODYNAMICS)

The pulmonary circulation is a low-pressure system compared with the systemic circulation, the mean pulmonary artery pressure at rest in normal subjects is about 15–20 mm Hg. At rest in the erect position in health the effect of gravity upon the distribution of blood from the pulmonary artery is marked. The amount of blood perfusing the upper lobes is less than that reaching the lower lobes because of the effects of gravity counteracting the filling pressure from the pulmonary artery. Increase in pulmonary artery pressure will result in a more even distribution of blood to all parts of the lungs. This happens in exercise in normal individuals through increase in cardiac output, and in a number of disease processes through changes in cardiac output or pulmonary vascular resistance. Similarly, any cause of increase in left atrial pressure will be transmitted to the pulmonary circulation resulting in increase in pulmonary capillary, pulmonary venous and pulmonary arterial pressures. Two other factors, *hypoxia* and *alveolar pressure*, may influence the distribution of pulmonary blood flow. Hypoxia causes pulmonary vasoconstriction due to a direct effect on the arterial smooth muscle. In any part of the lungs which becomes hypoxic as a result of reduced ventilation, active constriction of the pulmonary arterial circulation diverts blood away to better ventilated parts of the lungs. The pulmonary capillaries are compressible through the alveolar walls and if alveolar pressure is increased as a result of airways obstruction, blood will be redistributed away from these regions to less affected parts of the lungs. Not all alveoli perfused with blood are well ventilated, and any such alveoli will act as an effective 'shunt' for the pulmonary circulation i.e. blood passing through them will be returned to the left side of the heart still containing a large quantity of carbon dioxide and with a low oxygen content. This blood is sometimes referred to as the '*shunt*' and is increased in a variety of diseases.

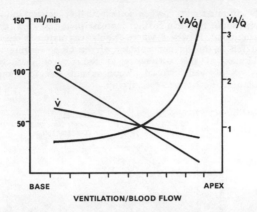

Fig. 8. Diagram of the distribution of ventilation, blood flow and ventilation—perfusion ratios in the normal upright lung. $\dot{Q}$, pulmonary blood flow. $\dot{V}$, ventilation. Note that at the apex, ventilation is greater relative to perfusion while at the bases perfusion exceeds ventilation. (Adapted from West J. B. (1977) *Ventilation, Blood Flow and Gas Exchange.* Oxford, Blackwell.)

VENTILATION—PERFUSION MATCHING

In the normal lung, ventilation and perfusion are not evenly matched throughout the lungs, but for the lungs as a whole, the distribution is relatively uniform (*Fig.* 8). Areas of the lungs in which ventilation is poor compared with perfusion will fail to contribute to respiratory gas exchange and will effectively constitute a '*shunt*' between the right and left sides of the heart so that blood passing through these alveoli will not be well oxygenated and will still contain venous quantities of carbon dioxide. Again, other alveoli which are well ventilated but poorly perfused will contribute to the *physiological dead space* and fail to contribute to gas exchange. Under resting conditions the quantity of carbon dioxide produced by the body will be constant and the carbon dioxide tension of alveolar air will depend only on the quantity of inspired air with which this carbon dioxide is mixed. If alveolar ventilation is high then the carbon dioxide tension of the air will be low, if ventilation is poor, then the carbon dioxide tension will rise. Because of the almost rectilinear shape of its dissociation curve, exchange of carbon dioxide is solely dependent on alveolar ventilation (*Fig.* 9). Oxygen exchange is more complex partly as a result of the more sigmoid shape of the oxygen dissociation curve (*Fig.* 9). Under normal conditions, blood leaving well-ventilated alveoli is almost completely saturated with oxygen so that further increase in ventilation of such alveoli cannot result in further increase in the oxygen content of the blood leaving them. However, where alveolar ventilation is reduced there is a resultant fall in the oxygen content of the blood leaving the affected alveoli. Because of this difference in the oxygen dissociation curve overventilation of well-perfused alveoli is not able to compensate for underventilation of other perfused alveoli.

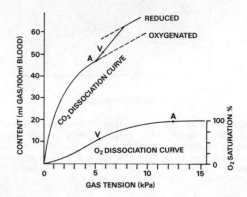

Fig. 9. The dissociation curve for oxygen and carbon dioxide of whole blood.
As the quantity of carbon dioxide carried by blood depends upon the degree of reduction of haemoglobin, the 'physiological' carbon dioxide dissociation curve lies between the curves for fully oxygenated and fully reduced haemoglobin. A and V are the normal values for arterial and mixed venous blood respectively.
Because the dissociation curve for carbon dioxide is steeper and straighter than that for oxygen, increase in ventilation of alveoli with high ventilation perfusion ratios can compensate for reduced excretion of carbon dioxide from alveoli with low ventilation—perfusion ratios. As the dissociation curve for oxygen is sigmoid in shape further increase in ventilation of alveoli which are already well ventilated and perfused cannot compensate by increased oxygen uptake for underventilated alveoli. (*After* Campbell E. J. M. Dickinson C. J. and Slater J. D. H. (1963) *Clinical Physiology,* 2nd ed. Oxford, Blackwell.)

CONTROL OF BREATHING

The depth and frequency of breathing are controlled by the respiratory centre which is a group of interconnected neurones in the medulla oblongata and pons (*Fig.* 10). Motor discharges from the respiratory centre are integrated at spinal level and carried thence by the phrenic and inter-costal nerves to the diaphragm and intercostal muscles. Afferent reflexes

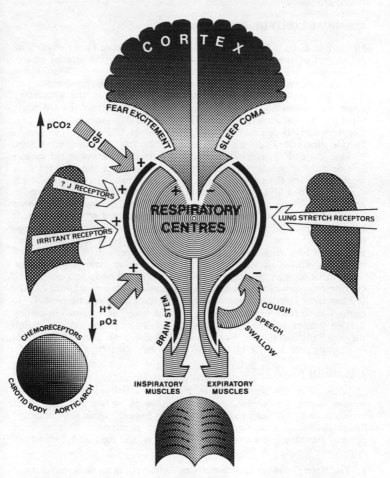

Fig. 10. Diagram of the respiratory centres and the more important factors controlling ventilation.

from a number of structures influence the output from the respiratory centre, but the major factors controlling ventilation are the carbon dioxide tension and hydrogen ion content of arterial blood and to a lesser extent its oxygen tension.

CHEMICAL CONTROL OF VENTILATION

The carbon dioxide tension of arterial blood is the major factor controlling the output of the respiratory centre, and, in health, the arterial carbon dioxide tension is maintained within narrow limits, about 5·2 kPa (40 mm Hg), an increase of only 0·1–0·2 kPa (1 or 2 mm Hg) provokes hyperventilation. Arterial carbon dioxide tension influences the respiratory centre by stimulating receptors on the surface of the medulla oblongata bathed by the cerebrospinal fluid (CSF), carbon dioxide may affect these receptors directly and also by diffusing into the CSF where the carbon dioxide liberates hydrogen ions which stimulate the chemoreceptors. Because the CSF is less well buffered than blood, changes in the carbon dioxide tension produce larger increases in hydrogen ion content than would occur for the same change in blood. This limitation of the buffering capacity of the CSF for hydrogen ions may account for delays in change in ventilatory pattern which occur after acid–base disturbances have been corrected in blood. In addition to the effects mediated by carbon dioxide tension in the CSF, the hydrogen ion content of the blood may also stimulate ventilation by effects on the carotid body and aortic arch chemoreceptors. Any rise in the hydrogen ion content of arterial blood stimulates ventilation. Changes in the arterial oxygen tension will increase the activity of the respiratory centre via the carotid body and aortic arch chemoreceptors when the arterial oxygen tension falls below about 8·0 kPa (60 mm Hg). Hypoxia also sensitizes the respiratory centre directly to changes in carbon dioxide tension so that when an increase in carbon dioxide tension is also accompanied by a fall in arterial oxygen tension the resultant increase in ventilation is greater than that which would accompany such a rise in carbon dioxide tension occurring alone.

THE HIGHER CENTRES

Impulses from the cerebral cortex affect the activity of the respiratory centres. Respiratory centre sensitivity is increased by fear and excitement and reduced during sleep and coma. Impulses from the brain stem interrupt breathing during coughing, swallowing and phonation. A number of afferent stimuli are carried in the vagus nerve and have an effect on the respiratory centres (*see Fig.* 10).

1. The Hering–Breuer (inflation reflex). Although in animals stretching of the lungs causes a reflex inhibition of inspiration, it is uncertain whether this reflex exists in man.

2. J-receptors. Juxtacapillary or J-receptors in the parenchyma of the lungs when stimulated increase ventilation. These receptors are believed to initiate the hyperventilation associated with pulmonary embolism and pulmonary oedema.

3. Irritant Receptors. These may be located in the distal bronchioles and are stimulated by irritant substances and local distortion. They again produce increase in ventilation and may be important in the reactions to irritant gases, asthma, pulmonary embolism and pneumonia.

4. Cough Receptors. There may be specific irritant receptors within the trachea and larger bronchi probably connected via the vagus nerve to the respiratory centre. Stimulation of these receptors initiates the cough reflex and may also result in an associated bronchoconstriction.

In addition to all these neurological controls of respiration, ventilation is probably also subject to influence through the respiratory centre by afferent stimuli from muscle tendons, joints and muscle spindles especially in the structures of the chest wall. These are important in the control of ventilation both at rest and during exercise.

OXYGEN TRANSPORT

Most of the oxygen carried in the blood is combined with haemoglobin in the red cells and a much smaller quantity is in simple solution in plasma. The oxygen combining capacity of haemoglobin is 1·34 ml per gram of haemoglobin and the amount of dissolved oxygen is about 0·003 ml/100 ml of blood/mm Hg oxygen gradient. The level of oxygen in blood can be measured as the tension or saturation. Direct measurement of oxygen tension with an oxygen electrode gives values in health between 10·6 and 13·3 kPa (about 80–100 mm Hg) and oxygen saturation varies between 95 and 98 per cent, but it can be increased to 100 per cent by breathing pure oxygen.

CARBON DIOXIDE TRANSPORT

Carbon dioxide is carried in blood in simple solution combined as bicarbonate ions and in combination with haemoglobin as carbamino compounds (*Fig.* 11). At the tissues carbon dioxide diffuses into the plasma and thence to the red cells before combining with water in the following reaction catalysed by the enzyme carbonic anhydrase present in red cells.

$$CO_2 + H_2O \rightleftharpoons H_2CO_3 \rightleftharpoons HCO_3^- + H^+.$$

Hydrogen ions are buffered by haemoglobin and bicarbonate ions diffuse back into the plasma to be replaced by chloride ions (the 'chloride shift').

The bulk of carbon dioxide in the blood is carried as bicarbonate in plasma. Thus red cells are important for the transport of carbon dioxide because (a) they contain carbonic anhydrase; (b) they contain haemoglobin for buffering and donating hydrogen ions; (c) reduced haemoglobin has a greater affinity for hydrogen ions than oxyhaemoglobin; and (d) reduced haemoglobin has a greater capacity for forming carbamino compounds.

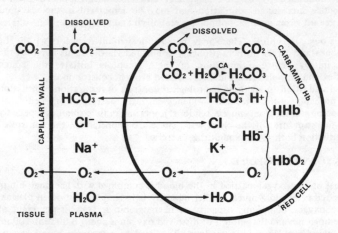

Fig. 11. Oxygen and carbon dioxide exchange between the red cells and the tissues at the systemic capillaries. At the pulmonary capillaries the reverse sequence of exchange occurs. (*By permission of Williams & Wilkins Co. Baltimore.*)

ACID–BASE CHANGES (*Table* 1)

The lungs are the main site of short-term acid–base regulation for the body, more long-term changes being effected by renal excretion and retention of ions. Alterations in ventilation bring about rapid changes in the excretion of carbon dioxide thus affecting the levels of carbon dioxide, bicarbonate and hydrogen ions in the blood. When the renal and respiratory compensatory mechanisms have not completely restored the acid–base balance this may be judged from knowledge of the arterial carbon-dioxide tensions, bicarbonate concentration and hydrogen ion content or pH measurement.

1. Metabolic Acidosis. This is present when the hydrogen ion content of blood is increased (pH reduced) and the bicarbonate content reduced.

Common causes include renal failure or diabetic ketosis through hydrogen ion accumulation and chronic diarrhoea or biliary fistulae causing loss of basic ions. Respiratory mechanisms are responsible for immediate compensation by hyperventilation with discharge of carbon dioxide and a resultant fall in bicarbonate and hydrogen ion content (rise in pH) of the blood.

2. Metabolic Alkalosis. This is present when the hydrogen ion content in the blood is reduced (pH increased) and the bicarbonate concentration is increased. Common causes include persistent vomiting, hypokalaemia or excessive bicarbonate administration. It may also result from inappropriate hyperventilation as may occur with anxiety. Respiratory compensation by hypoventilation produces a rise in hydrogen ion content (fall in pH) accompanied by a rise in bicarbonate concentration.

Table 1. Acid−base disturbance

	pH	$PaCO_2$	HCO_3	Causes
Metabolic acidosis	↓	↓	↓*	Diabetic ketosis, renal failure, chronic diarrhoea, biliary fistula
Metabolic alkalosis	↑	↑	↑*	Vomiting, hypokalaemia, excess bicarbonate therapy
Respiratory acidosis	↓	↑*	↑	Hypoventilation, e.g. respiratory failure, drug overdose
Respiratory alkalosis	↑	↓*	↓	Hyperventilation, e.g. liver failure, salicylate poisoning, head injury

↓ = reduction; ↑ = increase.
In each case * indicates the primary abnormality.

RESPIRATORY DISTURBANCES

Respiratory Acidosis. Any cause of respiratory failure may lead to an increase in carbon dioxide tension of the blood and tissues with a resultant increase in hydrogen ion (fall in pH) and bicarbonate content of blood. Renal mechanisms compensate by excretion of hydrogen ions and retention of bicarbonate ions.

Respiratory Alkalosis. May be caused by hyperventilation as in liver failure or poisoning with salicylates through stimulation of the respiratory centres by acid ions and following head injury. Arterial carbon dioxide tension is reduced and accompanied by a fall in hydrogen ion (rise in pH) and bicarbonate concentrations. Renal compensation leads to excretion of bicarbonate and retention of hydrogen ions.

Chapter 6

CLINICAL LUNG FUNCTION TESTS

Clinical lung function tests are valuable for defining the degree of abnormality in lung diseases and in serial assessment of patients as a guide to the progress of disease or the effects of treatment. It is uncommon for lung function tests to be essential in order to establish the diagnosis in respiratory diseases. The available tests may be divided into broad categories:

1. Tests of ventilatory function;
2. Tests of gas-exchanging function.

1. TESTS OF VENTILATORY FUNCTION

Lung Volumes. The total volume of gas in the lungs, conventionally measured at full inspiration i.e. total lung capacity (TLC), is conventionally subdivided into several fractions which are shown in *Fig.* 12. Population surveys of normal people have shown that the size of each of these subdivisions is significantly correlated with the height, age and sex of the individual.

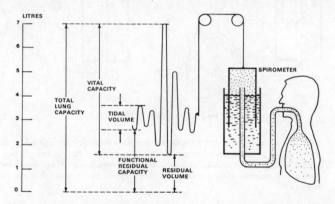

Fig. 12. The subdivisions of lung volume. N.B. functional residual capacity and residual volume cannot be measured by spirometery.

Static Lung Volumes. There are three methods by which total lung capacity and its subdivisions may be measured.

1. GAS DILUTION. An insoluble gas, usually helium, in known concentration is contained with air in a spirometer system. The

subject, wearing a nose clip, rebreathes with an airtight seal from the spirometer and at the same time oxygen is added to the spirometer mixture at a rate sufficient to replace that used by respiration. Within a few minutes when equilibration of the helium concentration between the spirometer and subject's lungs has occurred, because the total quantity of helium is unchanged and the volume of the spirometer and apparatus is known, it is possible by use of a simple equation to calculate the unknown volume of gas in the subject's lungs at the beginning of the procedure (*Fig.* 13).

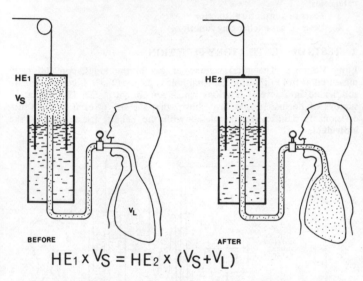

$$HE_1 \times V_S = HE_2 \times (V_S + V_L)$$

Fig. 13. Measurement of functional residual capacity by gas dilution methods. VS, volume of spirometer; VL, volume of the lung; HE_1 initial concentration of helium before rebreathing; HE_2 concentration of helium after equilibration by rebreathing with the gas in the lungs.

2. WHOLE BODY PLETHYSMOGRAPHY. The patient is seated in an airtight box (body plethysmograph) and pressure is measured continuously in the box (*Fig.* 14). A second manometer measures pressure at the patient's mouth. During inspiration enlargement of the thorax lowers the gas pressure within the chest but increases gas pressure in the plethysmograph. The change in intrathoracic pressure

is at any point in the respiratory cycle accompanied by equivalent but opposite change in plethysmograph pressure. In this method, lung volume is measured by interrupting airflow at some point in the respiratory cycle and then because the volume of the plethysmograph is known, and the pressures in the plethysmograph and chest are also known, the only unknown quantity is intrathoracic gas volume which can be calculated from a simple algebraic equation.

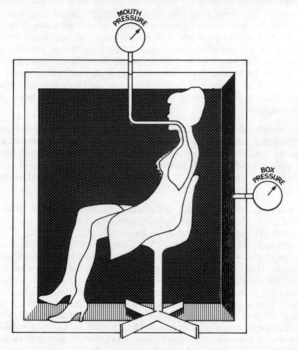

Fig. 14. Diagram of the whole body plethysmograph method for measuring functional residual capacity. The subject pants with low flow rates. Each change in intrathoracic pressure recorded by the mouth pressure manometer, produces an opposite change in box pressure. By application of Boyle's law lung volume can be calculated if the box volume is known.

3. RADIOLOGICAL METHODS. A number of simple techniques have been developed for deriving total lung volume from postero-anterior

and lateral chest X-rays by planimetry and more recently by computer methods. In these techniques, the lungs are treated as regular ellipsoids.

It is common for there to be some difference between lung volumes measured by plethysmograph and helium dilution as in the presence of marked airways obstruction or slowly ventilating spaces such as bullae and emphysematous areas, the gas-dilution methods will tend to underestimate total lung volume because the marker gas helium does not reach all parts of the lungs in the time available. In these circumstances (e.g. emphysema, bullae, severe airways obstruction in asthma or chronic bronchitis) the gas-dilution (helium) lung volume will be less than that measured by plethysmography which records total compressible gas volume. Similarly, in the presence of stiff lungs as in diffuse pulmonary fibrosis, radiological lung volume may be greater than that recorded in the plethysmograph because the increased stiffness makes the lungs less compressible and the radiological method fails to take account of the increased volume of tissue within the lungs.

Measurements of Forced Expiration. Airways obstruction is the commonest functional abnormality present in clinical lung disease e.g. it is the dominant functional abnormality in asthma and chronic bronchitis. The most widely used tests of airways obstruction are the forced expiratory measurements − forced vital capacity (FVC), forced expired volume in 1 second (FEV_1) and peak expiratory flow rate (PEFR).

Vital Capacity. Vital capacity is the maximum volume of air which can be expelled from the lungs after full inspiration and is usually measured by a spirometer. It can be reduced by restrictive defects, deformity of the chest and airways obstruction (*Fig.* 15). Generally three forced expiratory manoeuvres are made and the largest volume recorded for FVC and FEV_1 are taken. The FEV_1, the fraction of FVC expelled in the first second is reduced in obstructive diseases because of increased airways resistance. It will also be reduced in the presence of restrictive abnormalities but here the reduction is due to loss of lung volume rather than narrowing of the air airways, so that the normal ratio of FEV_1/FVC is maintained whereas in the presence of airways obstruction the FEV_1/FVC ratio is reduced. The degree of reversibility of airways obstruction may be assessed by recording FVC manoeuvres before and after inhalation of a bronchodilator aerosol. A very simple method which has proved invaluable for regular measurements at the bedside and assessment in out-patient clinics is measurement of peak expiratory flow rate (PEFR). This is the maximum flow over 10 microseconds at the beginning of forced expiration from full inspiration. It is usually measured with a Wright's peak flow meter although, recently, simpler and cheaper peak flow gauges have been introduced. Complex tests of lung function have indicated that measurements of FEV_1 and PEFR mainly reflect the dimensions of the larger airways in the lungs.

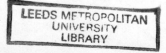

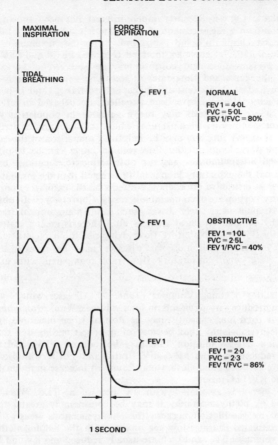

Fig. 15. Spirograms in a normal individual and patients with obstructive and restrictive ventilatory defects.

Airways Resistance. The total resistance of the respiratory airways (AWR) may be measured in the whole body plethysmograph but the additional information obtained from these more complex procedures is unwarranted in general clinical practice and offers no advantages over simple measurements of FEV_1, FVC and PEFR.

Flow-volume Curves. Recently much interest has been shown in tests where continuous measurement of flow rate is made during a full forced vital capacity inspiration and expiration. From the maximum expiratory flow-volume (MEFV) curve so obtained (*Fig.* 16) PEFR and FEV_1 can be derived. Pressure-dependent collapse may be observed in the expiratory limb of the curve and flow rates at low lung volumes near to residual volume e.g. after 50 per cent of vital capacity (MMF_{50}) and 75 per cent of vital capacity (MMF_{75}) have been expelled, are believed to reflect small airway calibre. Such tests may prove valuable in population screening programmes and other circumstances where the detection of early abnormalities of airway function may be helpful. Comparison of the expiratory and inspiratory loops of the flow-volume curve can be helpful. With generalized intrapulmonary airways obstruction (e.g. chronic bronchitis and asthma) the expiratory loop is more affected than the inspiratory loop (*Fig.* 16). In restrictive disorders the effects on the expiratory portion and inspiratory portion are of comparable severity. Conversely, with obstruction to the extrapulmonary larger airways such as the main bronchi, trachea and larynx (by tumours, tracheal stenosis etc.) there is greater restriction of inspiratory flow than expiratory flow giving rise to characteristic patterns (*Fig.* 16). Again, neuromuscular diseases may be revealed by their greater effect upon inspiratory flow rates compared with expiratory flow rates.

Abnormalities of Lung Volumes (*Table* 2). Diseases with airways obstruction produce varying effects on lung volumes. With *chronic obstructive bronchitis* total lung capacity may be normal when measured by wholebody plethysmography, but because of poor gas mixing due to airways obstruction the gas dilution TLC may be reduced. FEV_1 and FVC are usually reduced and the FEV_1/FVC ratio and PEFR will also be low. Airways obstruction and closure may cause an increase in residual volume (RV) and RV/TLC ratio.

Emphysema is associated with an increase in TLC. When TLC is measured by plethysmography it may be considerably greater than TLC measured by gas-dilution because the emphysematous areas of lung are poorly ventilated causing slow gas mixing with the helium method. The expired volumes FEV_1, and FVC are usually reduced and RV and RV/TLC ratio are increased. The loss of elastic recoil in emphysema leads to premature collapse of airways in expiration so that PEFR and FEV_1/FVC ratio will be low but although the airways collapse easily they may not be narrowed in themselves.

Patients with *asthma* may have normal lung volumes and airway function in remission but generally there is some increase in static volumes i.e. TLC, RV and RV/TLV are all increased. This is exaggerated in acute episodes and at such times TLC measured by plethysmography may be greater than TLC measured by gas dilution because of the effect of severe airways

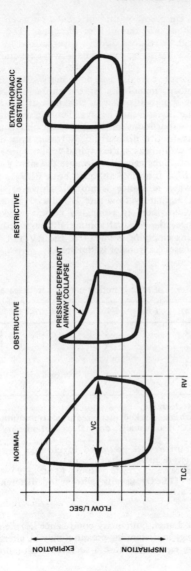

Fig. 16. Flow-volume loops. *Normal*, note that the peak inspiratory flow rate is greater than the peak expiratory flow rate. *Obstructive*, note that vital capacity is reduced and that the reduction in flow rates is greater in expiration than in inspiration. *Restrictive*, vital capacity again reduced, and flow rates are reduced in both expiration and inspiration, the normal relationship is preserved; extrathoracic obstruction, e.g. tracheal stenosis. Reduction in flow rates is greatest in inspiration.

obstruction on gas mixing. On recovery this difference between volume measured by the two methods will diminish or disappear. The expired volumes FEV_1 and FVC will be reduced during exacerbations of asthma and PEFR and FEV_1/FVC will also be low while airways resistance will be increased.

In *restrictive lung diseases* e.g. diffuse pulmonary fibrosis from sarcoidosis and pneumoconiosis, immobility of the thoracic cage as in kyphoscoliosis or ankylosing spondylitis or with weakness of the respiratory muscles in neuromuscular diseases such as myasthenia gravis, there will be a reduction in all the subdivisions of lung volume and total lung capacity. In general with restrictive diseases i.e. fibrosing lung diseases, neuromuscular and thoracic wall diseases, the expired volumes are reduced in parallel with the fall in total lung capacity. Because the airways are not obstructed the ratio FEV_1/FVC is normal although both FEV_1 and FVC are reduced. Similarly airways resistance is normal. However, because the lungs are smaller peak expiratory flow rate is reduced. In some of these diseases, especially where there is associated muscle weakness or stiffness of the thoracic cage, the residual volume although reduced in absolute volume because lung emptying is impaired, the RV/TLC ratio is increased. With fibrosing diseases gas transfer is impaired.

Table 2. Typical patterns of lung function changes in disease

	TLC	RV	FEV_1	FVC	FEV_1/FVC	TLCO
Asthma	1 ↑	1 ↑	↓	↓	↓	N[1] or ↓
Chronic bronchitis	N or ↑	↑	↓	↓	↓	N or ↓[2]
Emphysema	3 ↑	3 ↑	↓	↓	↓	3 ↓
Fibrosing diseases	↓	↓	↓	↓	N or ↑	↓

N = Normal; ↑ = increase; ↓ = decrease.
1. In severe episodes of asthma, marked increases in static volumes may occur. Gas transfer (TLCO) is usually normal except in very severe episodes.
2. Gas transfer (TLCO) is often well preserved in chronic obstructive bronchitis when there is severe airflow obstruction.
3. Combination of gross increase in static volume (TLC, RV) with reduction in gas transfer (TLCO) usually allows for differentiation between emphysema and asthma.

The Elastic Properties of the Lungs. Pulmonary compliance i.e. the change in lung volume for unit change in distending pressure, may be altered by a number of disease processes, especially those associated with pulmonary fibrosis where compliance will be reduced. Measurements of compliance are most usually made by a combination of intra-oesophageal pressure measurements with a balloon and catheter manometer system and simultaneous spirometric measurements of expired volume.

STATIC COMPLIANCE. Transpulmonary pressure i.e. the difference between oesophageal and mouth pressure, is recorded at a series of end-inspiratory lung volumes by interruption during a continuous vital capacity expiration. It is usual to express compliance measurements with reference to the lung volume at which they were made i.e. specific compliance (compliance divided by the lung volume). This is most meaningful at functional residual capacity. Compliance may be increased in emphysema because of loss of lung tissue and reduced by any disease associated with airways obstruction (e.g. chronic bronchitis and asthma) or with increased stiffness of the lungs from fibrosis (e.g. pulmonary fibrosis).

DYNAMIC COMPLIANCE, or compliance measured during continuous breathing, may be used to demonstrate minor abnormalities of the airways in the more peripheral parts of the lungs which are of uneven distribution. This is a complex test which is very unlikely to be of routine clinical use.

Distribution of Ventilation. In general two methods are used for testing the distribution of ventilation:

1. MULTIPLE BREATH METHOD. This is based on the principle that the time taken for an inhaled gas to achieve uniform concentration in all parts of the lungs will be longer if it is unevenly distributed. A spirometer containing an insoluble gas such as helium is used. The patient rebreathes from the spirometer system while a record is obtained of the falling concentration of helium in the system and the time taken to achieve equilibrium is compared with the time taken in normal individuals. The rate of change of helium concentration serves as an index of the evenness of distribution. In another method 100 per cent oxygen is breathed from a spirometer system and the change in nitrogen concentration in the system is used as the index of equality of ventilation.

2. SINGLE BREATH METHOD. This is based on the supposition that poorly ventilated aveoli will have a relatively high concentration of nitrogen and carbon dioxide and that their emptying will be delayed until the last part of expiration. In this method, either carbon dioxide or nitrogen concentration is recorded in expiration from total lung capacity. If the alveoli are evenly ventilated the nitrogen or carbon dioxide curve will be nearly flat. When there are many poorly ventilated alveoli the slope of the carbon dioxide or nitrogen curve will be increasingly steep (*Fig.* 17).

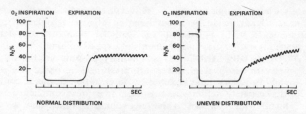

Fig. 17. The single breath nitrogen wash-out test. Nitrogen concentration is measured in the expired gas at the mouth. The subject takes a breath of pure oxygen to total lung capacity and then breathes out to residual volume. Normal distribution on the left. There is a rapid rise in nitrogen concentration as alveolar emptying begins and this is followed by the 'alveolar plateau' showing that nitrogen concentration throughout the lungs is even. Uneven distribution, the inspired oxygen has been unevenly distributed so that alveoli from different parts of the lungs will have a wide range of nitrogen concentrations. As the poorly ventilated parts empty last, there is a progressive rise in nitrogen concentration at the mouth.

2. MEASUREMENT OF GAS TRANSFER

Three factors govern the transfer of gases across the alveolar membrane: (1) Gas exchange can only occur where ventilated alveoli and perfused capillaries are in close proximity. Thus, if the airways are obstructed, the pulmonary vascular bed is occluded or the architecture of the alveoli is disrupted the surface for gas exchange is reduced and gas transfer will be reduced. (2) The distance across which gases must diffuse is also important, if the alveolar wall is thickened by increase in interstitial tissue or the presence of fluid, then gas transfer will be reduced. (3) The gas tension gradient across the alveolar membrane, if this is small the exchange of gas will be slow. In general, abnormalities of gas transfer, particularly of oxygen, are not usually due to obstruction to diffusion at the alveolar–capillary membrane ('alveolar–capillary block') but are caused by reduction in the effective surface area for gas exchange, uneven distribution of ventilation and perfusion or reduction in the number of red blood cells within the pulmonary capillaries or their haemoglobin content. For this reason, the term 'transfer factor' (TL) has been favoured for measurements of this capacity. The TL of the lung is expressed as mmol min^{-1} kPa^{-1} (ml of gas/minute/mm Hg). It is difficult to measure the mean capillary pressure of oxygen and for this reason carbon monoxide has become the standard gas used for measuring gas transfer because its diffusion rate and association constants with haemoglobin are similar to those of oxygen. As a result of its great affinity for haemoglobin and the fact that in normal individuals the capillary blood tension of carbon monoxide is zero, calculations are very much easier. Two methods are used for measuring carbon monoxide transfer (TLCO).

The Steady State Method. Here the subject breathes a gas mixture containing a low concentration of carbon monoxide for 1–2 min. This method can be used to measure gas transfer during exercise but in clinical practice the single breath method is easier to use.

The Single Breath Method. In this the patient takes a single vital capacity inspiration of a mixture of gases containing known concentrations of helium and carbon monoxide, breath-holds for 10 sec and then expires to residual volume. A sample of the expired air is taken in mid-expiration and

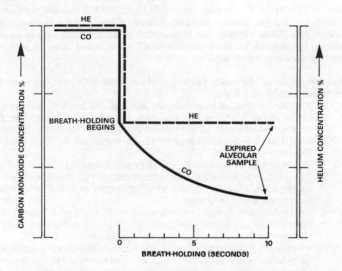

Fig. 18. Carbon monoxide transfer single breath method. The subject takes a vital capacity inspiration of a gas mixture containing helium and carbon monoxide, breath-holds for 10 sec, and then breathes out to residual volume. The diagram shows the helium and carbon monoxide traces at the mouth during expiration. If the gas mixture has been evenly distributed throughout the lungs, the helium trace will be horizontal. There is a progressive fall in carbon monoxide concentration due to absorption from the alveoli into the pulmonary capillary blood.

the concentrations of helium and carbon monoxide in this are measured. The dilution of the helium in the expired air compared to its concentration in the original gas mixture inhaled is used to calculate the alveolar volume (VA). This is a single-breath estimate of lung volume and gives the quantity of intrathoracic gas reached by the inspired mixture. If TLC is measured by another method e.g. plethysmography or radiological methods, VA can be subtracted from this to give volume of lung not reached by the gas mixture in the single breath. This difference is referred to as the 'trapped gas volume'. Calculation of carbon monoxide transfer is based upon the assumption that carbon monoxide is instantly diluted to the same degree as the helium and that the alveolar concentration falls exponentially to the expired level (*Fig.* 18). By integration, the rate of fall of concentration of carbon monoxide and the alveolar concentration of this gas can then be used to calculate the transfer factor (TLCO). The transfer factor (TLCO) may be divided by the alveolar volume (VA) to give the transfer coefficient (KCO) i.e. the gas transfer per unit volume of lung. This will correct for loss of lung tissue whether due to resection of lung, obstruction of a main airway by tumour or poor ventilation of an affected lobe or segment through airways obstruction.

Interpretation of Transfer Factor. Carbon monoxide transfer may be affected by the following:

1. Ventilation–perfusion imbalance. Much of the inspired gas may not reach perfused alveoli and this may be a factor in restrictive disorders, diseases with airways obstruction and where the pulmonary circulation has been affected by thrombo-embolic or other vascular diseases.
2. The thickness of the alveolar capillary membrane.
3. The surface area available for gas exchange e.g. this is reduced in emphysema, following resection of segments or lobes or destruction of lung tissue by disease.
4. The pulmonary capillary blood volume. This may be increased in heart failure and pulmonary haemorrhage giving increased values for gas transfer. It will be reduced in emphysema.
5. The haemoglobin concentration, thus carbon monoxide transfer will be reduced in the presence of anaemia and increased in the presence of polycythaemia.
6. The rate of reaction of carbon monoxide with haemoglobin.

Exercise Tests. Exercise tests can be useful for assessing cardiorespiratory function. At their simplest, assessment of the patient's capacity to walk on the level or up stairs may provide valuable information about the severity of breathlessness. By measuring minute ventilation, oxygen uptake, pulse rate with graded exercise loads, as with a bicycle ergometer or treadmill, allows more complex assessment of cardiorespiratory function but such tests require experience and skill. The reader is referred to reference works in the bibliography.

CLINICAL VALUE OF LUNG FUNCTION TESTS

Diagnosis. Respiratory failure may develop insidiously and often may only be apparent from arterial blood gas tension measurements. Where ventilatory capacity is most affected serial measurements of arterial carbon dioxide tension or mixed venous carbon dioxide tension by a rebreathing method are useful for the assessment of ventilation. With other forms of respiratory disability measurements of arterial oxygen tension are of value.

Cyanosis. Central cyanosis may be the result of uneven distribution of ventilation and perfusion, venous to arterial shunts, alveolar hypoventilation or any combination of these factors. Measurements of arterial oxygen saturation before and after breathing pure oxygen are invaluable. Failure to obtain 100 per cent saturation when breathing pure oxygen indicates a veno-arterial shunt.

Assessment of Medical Treatment

1. AIRWAYS OBSTRUCTION. In bronchial asthma or chronic airways obstruction the response to bronchodilators may be recorded by measurements of FEV_1 or PEFR before and after inhalation of the bronchodilator. The response to corticosteroids should be assessed by frequent measurements of FEV_1 or PEFR over the first 10–14 days of treatment. Similarly, in recovery from severe asthma diurnal variation in the severity of airflow obstruction is common and can be assessed with these measurements.

2. In restrictive lung diseases, such as sarcoidosis and fibrosing alveolitis, the effectiveness of corticosteroid therapy must be carefully assessed because of the euphoriant effects of such drugs leading to a false impression of improvement. At the outset where possible, full static and dynamic lung volumes should be recorded together with measurements of gas transfer and these should be repeated after a period of 4–6 weeks' treatment. If there has been no important change then these drugs may be regarded as ineffective.

Assessment for Operation. In spite of many attempts to obtain simple indices of suitability for operation, recognition of patients in the borderline group who may be likely to develop postoperative respiratory complications is difficult. The following may be useful.

1. An FEV_1 less than 35–40 per cent of predicted value for age and height suggests the patient is at risk.

2. Arterial carbon dioxide tension above 6·6 kPa (50 mm Hg) suggests the presence of alveolar hypoventilation.

3. An RV/TLC ratio greater than 50 per cent is abnormal.
4. Inability to perform simple exercise tests such as climbing a flight of stairs or walking comfortably on the flat.

Chapter 7

CHRONIC BRONCHITIS AND EMPHYSEMA

DEFINITIONS

It is common practice to group together chronic bronchitis and emphysema as conditions resulting in slowly progressive airways obstruction which is poorly reversible and associated with destruction of lung parenchyma. Many of these patients may have mucus hypersecretion but this is not invariable. Several attempts have been made to achieve working definitions for these diseases, the following are the most satisfactory: *Chronic bronchitis* (MRC, 1965) 'is a disease characterized by cough · productive of sputum on most days for at least three consecutive months for at least two successive years'. The sputum may be mucoid or mucopurulent and subdivisions of chronic bronchitis into simple, mucopurulent and obstructive have been adopted by some. This definition assumes that other causes for sputum production including bronchiectasis and tuberculosis have been excluded. *Emphysema* (CIBA Symposium, 1959) is defined in pathological terms as 'a disease in which there is increase beyond the normal size in the air spaces distal to the terminal bronchioles due to destruction of tissue and not simple overinflation'.

'Chronic bronchitis' has continued to be used without qualification to indicate a wide range of disability from one extreme of patients with regular production of small quantities of sputum without any abnormality of lung function to patients with severe airflow obstruction at the other extreme in whom little or no sputum is produced. Recent studies have suggested that mucus hypersecretion itself is a harmless condition which is not inevitably accompanied by progressive airway obstruction. Some patients may have clinical features predominantly of mucus hypersecretion and chronic airways obstruction with little or no evidence of emphysema while others may present with gross emphysema and little or no mucus hypersecretion. However, in most studies the majority of patients have belonged to a heterogeneous middle group in which the features of mucus hypersecretion, airways obstruction and emphysema are present together in varying proportions. One detailed study (Fletcher et al., 1976) produced results which suggest that there may be two distinct processes linked to susceptibility to smoking and other forms of air pollution. On the one hand the tendency to mucus hypersecretion and on the other the development of airflow obstruction (*Fig.* 19).

EPIDEMIOLOGY

Very large variations in mortality rates for bronchitis between different countries are striking, Britain has the highest mortality rate for this disease.

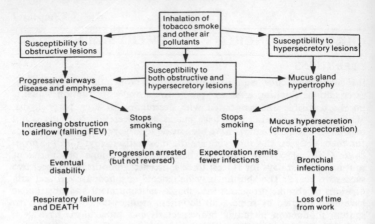

Fig. 19. Schematic representation of the 'natural histories' of airways obstruction and mucus hypersecretion (Taken from Fletcher et al. (1976) *Natural History of Chronic Bronchitis and Emphysema.* London, Oxford University Press.)

In studies in Britain using the above definition the prevalence in men was 8 per cent and in women 3 per cent of the population. Bronchitis is also the largest single cause of loss of work in Britain.

PATHOLOGY

Chronic Bronchitis (*Fig.* 20). There is hypertrophy of mucus-secreting glands of the bronchial tree and a great increase in the number of goblet cells, especially in the bronchioles. The causes of airways obstruction include excessive mucus, the encroachment on the lumen on the glandular structures (*see Fig.* 20), a variable increase in the quantity of bronchial smooth muscle and in advanced cases foci of collapse, inflammation and scarring scattered irregularly throughout the lungs with intervening areas of centrilobular emphysema.

Emphysema. Two main kinds are recognized to be of importance in connection with chronic airways obstruction (*Fig.* 21).

1. CENTRILOBULAR (or centri-acinar) where dilatation and destruction of the small airways at the level of the respiratory bronchioles leaves most of the alveoli in each respiratory lobule unaffected.

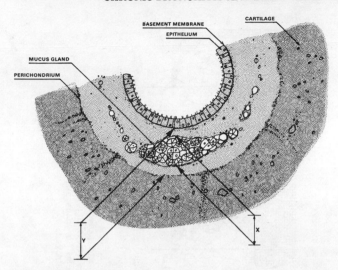

Fig. 20. Diagram of a cross-section of the bronchial wall in chronic obstructive bronchitis showing the 'Reid index'. In the normal bronchus the area (x) occupied by mucus glands is less than one-third of the width of the submucosal area (y), i.e. x/y is 0·3 or less. In chronic obstructive bronchitis it is two-thirds or more, i.e. x/y = 0·6. This is the 'Reid index'.

2. PANACINAR OR PAN-LOBULAR (idiopathic, primary, essential or cryptogenic), where there is widespread dilatation and destruction of most of the alveoli within many respiratory lobules. Both types of emphysema may be seen in the same individual. In association with chronic bronchitis the commonest type of emphysema to be seen is centrilobular. Panacinar emphysema may occur at any age but tends to develop early (before 50 years) with a familial incidence. This type has been linked with deficiency of alpha-1-antitrypsin in peripheral blood. This is a protein which inactivates proteolytic enzymes such as leucocyte collagenase and elastase. Deficiency of this enzyme is inherited as a recessive gene and about 1 in 2500 individuals in Britain shows gross deficiency of alpha-1-antitrypsin and greatly increased liability to pulmonary emphysema especially in the lower lobes.

   At least two other forms of emphysema are recognized histologically.

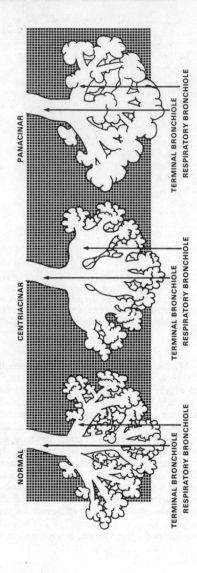

Fig. 21. Diagram of centri-acinar and panacinar emphysema. In centri-acinar emphysema the tissue destruction is mainly around the terminal and respiratory bronchioles. In panacinar emphysema, alveoli throughout the acinus are destroyed.

3. PERIACINAR (PARASEPTAL) EMPHYSEMA. At the edge of the acinus where it is bounded by connective tissue enlarged air spaces develop. This type is thought not to be directly associated with airways obstruction but may lead to the formation of bullae or spontaneous pneumothorax.
4. SCAR (IRREGULAR) EMPHYSEMA. This occurs perhaps as a result of lung injury from a variety of causes and is irregularly distributed within acini. It is not necessarily associated with airways obstruction.

AETIOLOGY AND PATHOGENESIS

A number of factors have been linked with the incidence of chronic bronchitis.

Cigarette smoking is a major factor in the development of chronic bronchitis and emphysema, so that severe breathlessness and sputum production occurring in a non-smoker should raise the possibility of an alternative diagnosis.

Atmospheric pollution. High prevalence and mortality rates for bronchitis have been linked with increasing urbanization and seasonal peaks of mortality correspond with peaks of air pollution.

Occupation. Prevalence and mortality are higher in workers in industries where irritant gases and dusts are common, and striking differences in mortality rates for different socio-economic groups have been recorded e.g. mortality rate in social class V (unskilled manual workers) is 6- or 8-fold higher than in classes I and II (professional and administrative workers).

Infection. It is unlikely that chronic bronchitis is mainly propagated by infection. Individuals with mucus hypersecretion may develop temporary increase in airways obstruction with mucopurulent sputum resulting from infection with *H. influenzae* or *S. pneumoniae* but on recovery there is no permanent deterioration of lung function. The rate of deterioration in such individuals is no greater than that found in others who do not develop infections.

Genetic Factors. Apart from the rare but well-recognized link between panacinar emphysema and alpha-1-antitrypsin deficiency no other inherited factors associated with susceptibility to chronic bronchitis or emphysema have been identified.

Two previous models for the pathogenesis of chronic bronchitis were proposed.
1. *Infection.* It was believed that lower respiratory tract infections resulted in damage to the airways with hypertrophy of mucous glands leading to airways obstruction and further progression. This model now seems unlikely to be correct.

2. *Hyper-reactivity*. The presence of bronchial hyper-reactivity, similar to that seen in asthma, has been thought to be a prerequisite for the development of chronic bronchitis. Present opinion in the UK and USA does not favour this hypothesis as a major causative factor for most patients.

RADIOLOGY

In patients with advanced chronic bronchitis a simple postero-anterior chest X-ray may show no abnormality but often there is evidence of overinflation with low flat diaphragms, elongation of the cardiac shadow and prominence of the hilar vessels due to enlargement of the proximal pulmonary arteries. In patients with extensive panacinar emphysema increased radiolucency in the lung fields may be visible. When right heart failure develops cardiac enlargement and upper lobe venous distension become prominent features on chest X-ray.

FUNCTIONAL ABNORMALITY

The most important feature is generalized airways obstruction. The factors contributing to this include increased secretions, mainly mucus, within the airways, thickening of the bronchial mucous membrane by hypertrophy of mucous glands and oedema, increase in smooth muscle tone, distortion of peripheral airways by destruction and fibrosis and emphysema. Simple measurements of FEV_1, PEFR and FVC are most useful. Once the disease is established all will be reduced and the FEV_1/FVC ratio will be low. Some patients may show a reversible component to the airways obstruction but if this amounts to more than 10 or 20 per cent it is likely that they have coincident asthma. The lungs are usually overinflated with increase in TLC, RV and RV/TLC ratio. Diffusing capacity for carbon monoxide (TLCO) is not seriously affected until advanced chronic bronchitis is present. In emphysema the most striking features are gross overinflation with marked reduction of carbon monoxide diffusing capacity. At rest, except in advanced disease, arterial blood gas tensions may be normal but patients with chronic bronchitis show a tendency for carbon dioxide retention and hypoxia because of chronic underventilation. Those in whom emphysema is widespread often retain normal sensitivity to carbon dioxide and when hypoxia develops they show a compensatory hyperventilation. Only with very advanced disease do such patients develop carbon dioxide retention.

CLINICAL FEATURES OF CHRONIC BRONCHITIS AND EMPHYSEMA

Characteristic features are productive cough with wheezing and breathlessness but patients may have little sputum but marked airways obstruction. There is usually a history of cigarette smoking and early morning cough. Breathlessness varies considerably in severity and may suddenly become marked following an exacerbation with or without infection. There is often a poor correlation between the degree of breathlessness and the severity of the airways obstruction as measured. The severity of exercise limitation is a useful prognostic feature, patients whose walking capacity is reduced on level ground have only a 60 per cent chance of surviving 5 years. Sputum may be mucoid but purulent during exacerbations.

Patients have been classified into two polar groups according to their tendency to develop carbon dioxide retention and underventilation but the majority belong to a confused middleground. *'Pink puffers' (Type A)* are usually thin, severely breathless at rest and produce little sputum. Although they develop marked arterial oxygen desaturation with effort they remain normally sensitive to carbon dioxide and only show hypercapnia as a pre-terminal event. In these patients peripheral oedema or right heart failure develops late and usually heralds death within a year. Such patients show severe airways obstruction by conventional tests (FEV_1/FVC and PEFR), increased total lung capacity and reduced diffusing capacity for carbon monoxide. Chest X-ray usually shows evidence of panacinar emphysema. *'Blue Bloater' (Type B)*. This type of patient is commoner, usually obese with copious sputum production and may have frequent exacerbations often with infected sputum. These patients show a tendency to underventilation and insensitivity to carbon dioxide so that they are commonly hypoxaemic with hypercapnia, especially during acute exacerbations. They may have secondary polycythaemia and renal bicarbonate retention leading to the development of peripheral oedema in the absence of right heart failure. Compared to type A patient's lung function tests in type B patients may show less severe airways obstruction and total lung capacity, residual volume and carbon monoxide diffusing capacity are nearer normal. There are often no signs suggestive of the presence of emphysema on chest X-ray.

Clinical Signs. Noisy breath sounds may be audible at a distance from the patient and expiration may be prolonged through pursed lips. Inspiration may be aided by contraction of the accessory muscles of respiration including the infrathyroid strap muscles. The wide swings of intrathoracic pressure associated with airways obstruction cause indrawing of the supraclavicular fossae and intercostal spaces during inspiration with jugular venous distension on expiration. Chest expansion may be poor with an increase in the anteroposterior diameter of the chest due to overinflation making the apex beat impalpable and reducing the areas of cardiac and liver dullness. In type A patients breath sounds may be very quiet or inaudible through the stethoscope but in type B patients wheezes and crackles are usually present. When right ventricular hypertrophy develops there may be a parasternal heave and a loud pulmonary second sound, but again these may be masked by overinflation.

INVESTIGATIONS

During exacerbations with infection there may be a polymorph leucocytosis and raised ESR. Persistent hypoxia may lead to a secondary polycythemia.

Sputum Examination. In patients with sputum, leucocytes may be present between exacerbations and where there is an asthmatic component eosinophils may also be found in the sputum. *H. influenzae* and *S. pneumoniae* are the most common organisms to be isolated from sputum cultures.

Chest X-ray. This often appears normal in chronic bronchitis but in patients with emphysema hyperinflation causes low flat diaphragms, a long thin heart and increase of the space anterior to the heart in the lateral film. Attenuation and narrowing of peripheral vessels and bullae may be recognized.

Pulmonary Function Tests. FEV_1, FVC and PEFR are usually reduced, with severe bronchitis the FEV_1 is usually less than 1 litre and the FEV_1/FVC ratio 30 per cent or less. A little improvement may follow inhalation of a bronchodilator aerosol and some patients may improve after inhalation of atropine. Most patients have an increased RV and RV/TLC ratio and in those patients with emphysema TLC is usually grossly increased. Carbon monoxide diffusing capacity is severely reduced with emphysema but nearer normal in uncomplicated chronic bronchitis.

Blood Gas Analysis. In 'Pink Puffers' (Type A) at rest the arterial oxygen tension may be normal with a normal or low carbon dioxide tension but on effort arterial desaturation usually develops. In 'Blue Bloaters' (Type B) patients with chronic bronchitis and little emphysema the arterial oxygen tension may be reduced at rest and the arterial carbon dioxide tension increased at rest and especially with exercise or during acute exacerbations. A compensatory increase in serum bicarbonate concentration accompanies this carbon dioxide retention.

DIFFERENTIAL DIAGNOSIS

Bronchiectasis. A history of chronic cough, breathlessness and sputum production due to bronchiectasis may at first be mistaken for chronic bronchitis, especially in younger patients. The perennial nature of the cough beginning early in life following measles, whooping cough or pneumonia will make the differentiation from chronic bronchitis but some patients with bronchiectasis, especially affecting the upper lobes may only produce sputum during acute infective episodes. Where doubt remains and plain X-rays are not characteristic the use of bronchograms may be necessary.

Bronchial Carcinoma. Bronchial carcinoma and chronic bronchitis commonly occur in the same patient because of their connection with cigarette smoking. In most instances obvious radiological abnormality will be present with carcinoma of the bronchus. Suspicious features are haemoptysis, finger clubbing or unresolved pneumonia in middle-aged smokers.

Tuberculosis. This should still be considered, especially in Asian immigrants, presenting with a history of cough and breathlessness. Usually the chest X-ray abnormality is typical of tuberculosis and will indicate the need for further investigations. Rarely endobronchial tuberculosis may present as productive cough with a normal chest X-ray.

MANAGEMENT

Long-term Treatment

GENERAL MEASURES. Commonly patients with chronic bronchitis and emphysema are unaware that cigarette smoking is linked with their disability. For most patients vigorous encouragement to abandon smoking is justified and smoking advisory clinics and hypnosis may sometimes be helpful. In patients with pre-terminal disease it is often inhuman to insist that they stop smoking. Obese patients should be encouraged to lose weight and to improve their exercise tolerance by simple physical training exercises such as progressive stair climbing or walking on the flat to help to increase their capacity for general activities. Breathing exercises may also be helpful.

ANTIBIOTICS. In patients with productive cough the duration of infective episodes and the associated temporary worsening of respiratory function may be avoided or reduced by short courses of antibiotics started at the first sign of respiratory tract infection. Suitable antibiotics include oxytetracycline, co-trimoxazole, ampicillin and amoxycillin in conventional doses for 5–7 days.

BRONCHODILATORS. Although less effective than in asthma, bronchodilators should be tried in patients with chronic bronchitis. Check that pressurized sympathomimetic aerosols are inhaled effectively and of oral preparations phyllocontin (Aminophylline) or salbutamol (Ventolin) tablets are most suitable.

MUCOLYTIC AGENTS. No convincing evidence exists that these drugs are important in the management of chronic bronchitis but some patients feel that it is easier to raise their sputum when treated with Bisolvon. Inhalation of steam vapours or Friar's Balsam may be very effective in acute exacerbations.

TREATMENT OF PERIPHERAL OEDEMA. A mild diuretic to reduce oedema gives improvement in some patients with chronic bronchitis. One of the thiazides with potassium supplements is suitable. With cor pulmonale and severe cardiac failure in the absence of atrial flutter or fibrillation digoxin is unlikely to be helpful and may easily induce other dysrhythmias.

COUGH SUPPRESSANTS. Where possible avoid cough suppressants in treating chronic bronchitis as they may lead to sputum retention and acute exacerbations of respiratory failure. Where cough is particularly troublesome one of the non-opiate central antussives such as dextromethorphan may be safest.

CORTICOSTEROIDS. These are not generally effective in chronic bronchitis and emphysema except where an asthmatic component is present. In patients with sputum or blood eosinophilia or significant reversibility of FEV_1, FVC or PEFR a trial of prednisolone 40 mg daily for 10–14 days should be assessed with frequent measurements of PEFR and walking distance to detect true and placebo responses. It is often difficult to select which patients are likely to respond to corticosteroids and it is probably justified to give a trial to all patients with severe airways obstruction provided that a system of objective assessment is used.

OXYGEN AT HOME. Patients with advanced disease may be helped by a supply of oxygen at home especially for climbing stairs, dressing and other short activities. Oxygen can be supplied in large cylinders from which a small portable apparatus can be refilled. The value of prolonged oxygen therapy for reducing pulmonary hypertension in chronic bronchitis is being assessed.

Treatment of Acute Respiratory Failure. The aim of treatment is to clear secretions and improve ventilation without enhancing carbon dioxide retention. Admission to hospital is usually necessary for frequent simple physiotherapy and controlled oxygen therapy.

Initial Assessment. A careful history, usually from a relative, is necessary to find how rapid deterioration has been and what the patient's previous state was like. A chest X-ray may show areas of consolidation or occasionally a pneumothorax which has caused sudden worsening of respiratory failure. Measurement of carbon dioxide tension in mixed venous blood by the rebreathing method or in arterial blood by puncture is important to assess the danger of carbon dioxide retention. Knowledge of the arterial oxygen tension is of lesser importance but may be helpful. Blood urea and serum electrolytes will be abnormal with dehydration or renal failure and the plasma bicarbonate level will be raised in compensated chronic respiratory failure. Sputum culture may be helpful although the majority of exacerbations occurring outside hospital due to infection are caused by *H. influenzae* or *S. pneumoniae*. Patients should be nursed sitting up in bed and encouraged to cough and take deep breaths. Such simple physio-therapy given by medical or nursing staff can be very effective and is to be preferred to professional physiotherapy at infrequent intervals.

Oxygen. Those patients admitted to hospital with exacerbations of chronic bronchitis and emphysema are often profoundly hypoxaemic. Preservation of the hypoxic drive to respiration is vital and injudicious oxygen therapy which removes this drive may lead to progressive carbon dioxide retention and coma if sensitivity to carbon dioxide is impaired. Before treatment is begun a measurement of arterial or mixed venous carbon dioxide tension is invaluable. If this is normal treatment may be begun with 28 per cent oxygen but if the initial arterial carbon dioxide tension is 8·0 kPa (60 mm Hg) or more the inspired oxygen concentration should not be greater than 24 per cent. Once treatment has begun close observation of the level of consciousness is important and the mixed venous or arterial pCO_2 should be remeasured. If the pCO_2 has not risen and drowsiness does not occur the inspired oxygen concentration may be increased at intervals provided that measurements confirm that progressive hypercapnia is not occurring.

Respiratory Stimulants. Where possible regular encouragement to cough and take deep breaths alone should be used. If this is not effective nikethamide is best given by intermittent i.m. injections of 2 ml (25 per cent solution). Doxapram, a short acting respiratory stimulant, is recom-mended for continuous i.v. infusion at a rate of 1–2 mg per minute, caution being necessary. *Avoidance of sedatives* for noisy, confused patients is essential as these are usually the effects of hypoxia and hypercapnia.

Treatment of Heart Failure. Diuretics may be valuable and frusemide 40 mg by i.v. injection is good initial treatment, thereafter bendrofluazide or chlorthiazide should be given daily. For severe intractable cor pulmonale a combination of spironolactone and amiloride is sometimes effective when other diuretics fail.

Failure of Improvement or Deterioration. If these measures fail to produce improvement assisted ventilation may be considered to improve oxygen-ation and help remove secretions. *Careful assessment of the patient's previous state is advisable.* The ideal patient is one in whom this is the first severe exacerbation of respiratory failure, who is under 60 years of age and who has previously been able to work or lead a useful life at home with the support of a loving family. Any departure from these criteria is one less indication for assisted ventilation. Expert help is needed to administer intermittent positive-pressure ventilation. Mild sedation should be used and the aim should be to achieve arterial oxygen tensions of the order of 8–14 kPa (60–105 mm Hg). Where the arterial carbon dioxide tension has been raised this should be allowed to fall slowly as sudden changes may cause cerebral vasoconstriction.

Chapter 8

BRONCHIECTASIS AND CYSTIC FIBROSIS

BRONCHIECTASIS

Definition. Bronchiectasis is chronic dilatation of bronchi with impaired drainage of bronchial secretions usually with persistent infection of the affected lobe or segment. Bronchiectasis usually starts in childhood but the onset can occur in adult life. The incidence has fallen, probably as a result of the use of effective antibiotic therapy for chest infections in children.

Aetiology and Pathogenesis
1. CONGENITAL. In Kartagener's syndrome dextrocardia and sinusitis are associated with bronchiectasis, possibly with ciliary abnormalities. Sequestrated lung segments and bronchomalacia may be associated with bronchiectasis.
2. IMMUNODEFICIENCY. Congenital or acquired hypogamma-globulinaemia may be complicated by the development of bronchiectasis.
3. CYSTIC FIBROSIS. As a result of bronchial obstruction by mucus with secondary bacterial infection most patients with cystic fibrosis develop bronchiectasis.
4. BRONCHIAL OBSTRUCTION. Obstruction of a bronchus by tumour, inhaled foreign bodies or mucus plugs may be followed by distal secondary infection with damage to bronchi and subsequent dilatation and distortion to give bronchiectasis.
5. PERTUSSIS (WHOOPING COUGH), MEASLES, TUBERCULOSIS AND PNEUMONIA. Either in childhood or adult life may be complicated by subsequent bronchiectasis due to damage to bronchial walls.
In all examples so far given the more distal bronchi are usually affected. In contrast
6. ALLERGIC BRONCHOPULMONARY ASPERGILLOSIS. Causes an unusual form of bronchiectasis affecting more proximal medium-sized bronchi.

Whatever the initial cause, the inflammatory processes result in damage to the bronchial walls with destruction of cartilage and a change from the normal ciliated epithelium to a more columnar or cuboidal form. The bronchial mucus gland content is increased and the bronchial circulation may show widespread anastomoses with varicosities. Bronchiectasis may be localized or widespread and the left lung is affected most commonly but about half of all cases are bilateral. Because of the anatomical form of the bronchial tree and the effects of gravity the lobes most often affected are the lower lobe and middle lobe on the right and the lingula and lower lobe on the left.

Bacteriology. Initial infection is usually with a mixture of organisms, *H. influenzae, S. pneumoniae* and *S. aureus* being commonest. With established disease anaerobic organisms are usually present in addition and *E. coli, Proteus, P. aeruginosa* and *K. pneumoniae* may also be found.

Clinical Features

1. ONSET. Symptoms usually begin in childhood, often with a recognizable respiratory illness such as whooping cough, measles or pneumonia.
2. COUGH. This is usually present throughout the year but is made worse by respiratory infections.
3. SPUTUM. This is usually purulent and copious, 100 ml or more may be produced daily. Paroxysms of coughing occur particularly on rising after sleep when the change of posture disturbs the accumulated secretions.
4. HAEMOPTYSIS. Caused by bleeding from bronchopulmonary arterial anastomoses; is very common especially with exacerbations of infection. It may occasionally cause anaemia but is rarely life-threatening.
5. DYSPNOEA. It is usually only present with widespread bilateral bronchiectasis.
6. WHEEZE. This may be prominent if several bronchi are affected.
7. SINUSITIS AND NASAL POLYPS. Are present in about 70 per cent of cases.
8. SYSTEMIC SYMPTOMS. Extensive bronchiectasis with copious purulent sputum may cause malaise, anorexia, weight loss and fever. In children this may result in failure to thrive with stunting of growth. Previously bronchiectasis was a common cause of amyloidosis.

Physical Signs. Coarse crackles and wheezes are usually audible over the affected segments or lobes. Signs of consolidation and collapse may be present when an acute episode of infection is superimposed. Finger clubbing is common especially when central cyanosis is present or extensive sepsis has persisted for years.

Investigations

1. CHEST X-RAY. This can be normal but usually shows crowding and haziness of the vascular markings in the affected areas and thickened bronchial walls may also be visible. Cyst-like shadows, sometimes with fluid levels, are common.
2. SPUTUM. *Examination and cultures for micro-organisms, including anaerobes and acid-fast bacilli.* This is particularly valuable during acute exacerbations as the sensitivities of the organisms can be assessed.

3. BRONCHOGRAPHY. This will show contrast medium pooling in dilated bronchi. It is unnecessary as a routine investigation but it is essential to define the extent of the disease if surgery is planned. Occasionally it may be helpful in planning correct postural drainage.
4. BRONCHOSCOPY. This should be considered in children and young adults to exclude the presence of a foreign body or benign tumour such as an adenoma.
5. SWEAT TEST. To exclude the presence of cystic fibrosis.
6. SERUM IMMUNOGLOBULIN LEVELS. These should be measured to identify the occasional patient who has an immunodeficiency in whom treatment with the gammaglobulin may be helpful.

Management

1. MEDICAL. This is usually successful in most cases and consists of adequate postural drainage and effective antibiotic therapy. The patient should be taught the positions to adopt to drain the affected segments or lobes by using gravity. It must become a daily routine each morning, preferably with chest percussion given by a family member. In severe cases and during acute exacerbations postural drainage and percussion should be repeated in the evening.

Antibiotics for the control of acute exacerbations must be effective against *H. influenzae*, *S. aureus* and *S. pneumoniae*. Cultures should be made of fresh sputum but treatment may be started with amoxycillin 500 mg 6-hourly before the results are available. Where staphylococci are isolated flucloxacillin 500 mg 6-hourly should be added and if anaerobic organisms are present metronidazole 800 mg 8-hourly is the treatment of choice.

Generally it is advisable to give patients a reserve supply of amoxycillin to keep in readiness for prompt treatment of exacerbations but continuous antibiotic treatment should be avoided as this tends to permit the emergence of *P. aeruginosa* as a persistent pathogen. Where this is a problem an intensive 10-day course of intravenous carbenicillin 5 g 6-hourly and gentamicin 2 mg/kg 8-hourly may occasionally eradicate this organism but usually only produces temporary suppression of its growth.

In patients with excessive copious sputum long-term treatment with low doses of tetracycline may sometimes be helpful.
2. SURGICAL. Indications:
   a. Failed medical treatment in young patients and where
   b. A single segment or lobe of a lung is affected and overall lung function is sound.
   c. Occasionally resection of a segment may be indicated for severe haemoptysis although the disease may occupy more than one segment or lobe. In this case the bleeding segment identified at bronchoscopy is excised. More recently success has been obtained

by planned intravascular obstruction of the relevant blood vessel carried out with radiological control.

Differential Diagnosis

1. ACUTE BRONCHITIS. Recurrent attacks, especially in childhood, can usually be differentiated from bronchiectasis because of the absence of cough and sputum between acute episodes and the smaller volume of sputum produced.
2. CHRONIC BRONCHITIS. Here cough and sputum usually with wheezing start later in life. The history and the smaller volume of sputum produced are usually helpful in making the distinction.
3. PNEUMONIA. This is unlikely to be confused with bronchiectasis because of the short history.
4. PULMONARY TUBERCULOSIS AND BRONCHIAL CARCINOMA. These may cause chronic cough and haemoptysis but can usually be differentiated from bronchiectasis by a careful history, chest X-ray, sputum bacteriology and cytology.

Complications of Bronchiectasis

1. Chronic bronchitis.
2. Pneumonia and pleurisy with recurrent infection.
3. Empyema.
4. Lung abscess.
5. Brain abscess.
6. Severe haemoptysis.
7. Secondary amyloidosis.
8. Respiratory failure and cor pulmonale.

Prevention. Prompt treatment of acute lower respiratory tract infections in children with antibiotics and physiotherapy, together with immunization against whooping cough and measles, have helped to reduce the incidence and prevalence of the disease.

CYSTIC FIBROSIS (Fibrocystic Disease of the Pancreas; Mucoviscidosis)

This is an inherited disorder of exocrine glands characterized by hypertrophy and hyperplasia of mucus-secreting glands, a high concentration of sodium chloride in sweat and in 95 per cent of patients pancreatic insufficiency causing malabsorption. The disease is inherited by an autosomal recessive gene, the incidence of affected individuals who are homozygous for the abnormal gene is 1 in 2500–3000 live births and the incidence of heterozygotes who are asymptomatic carriers is 1 in 25 live births.

Pathology

THE PANCREATIC LESION. The exocrine tissue of the pancreas atrophies but the ducts remain as isolated cysts, hence the name. This pancreatic failure results in malabsorption with steatorrhoea.

THE PULMONARY LESION. Excess mucus is produced and the small bronchi and bronchioles which are normal at birth become blocked by mucus. Subsequent destructive changes lead to the development of bronchiectasis.

Clinical Features. The majority of patients are recognized during childhood because of recurrent chest infections, symptoms of malabsorption and failure to thrive. About 10 per cent of affected children present with meconium ileus shortly after birth. As the disease advances breathlessness on exertion develops and this leads to respiratory failure and eventual death.

Diagnosis. In many cases the diagnosis is readily recognized from the association of recurrent chest infections and pancreatic failure. The diagnosis is confirmed by measurement of the sodium chloride concentration in sweat. This is raised although it may be normal in some affected adults.

Management
1. DIET. A low-fat diet is advisable with supplements of fat-soluble vitamins. Pancreatic supplements are given as powders or capsules (e.g. Pancrex, Nutrizyme and Cotazym).
2. PULMONARY LESION
   a. *Postural Drainage with Percussion* must be carried out twice daily throughout life. The clearance of secretions can be helped by the use of bronchodilator aerosols before physiotherapy is carried out.
   b. *Treatment of Infection.* In early childhood *S. aureus* is the usual organism found in sputum and it is common practice to give an antistaphylococcal antibiotic (e.g. cloxacillin or flucloxacillin) continuously for the first two years of life. Later *H. influenzae* replaces *S. aureus* as the main pathogen and in those patients who survive into the third and fourth decades *P. aeruginosa* tends to be the dominant pathogen. Antibiotic therapy should always be given at times of upper respiratory tract infections or exacerbations of sputum production and amoxycillin or oxytetracycline with cloxacillin would be suitable combinations to use. Where anaerobic organisms are present metronidazole should be added and if *P. aeruginosa* is found carbenicillin and gentamicin should be given in combination for 10 days as directed for the treatment of bronchiectasis. Bronchodilators by aerosol are helpful to relieve airways obstruction. Prophylactic polyvalent influenza vaccine should be given each winter and immunization against whooping cough and measles should be carried out in infancy.

Complications

DIABETES MELLITUS. This develops in some adult patients but it usually responds to treatment with diet and oral hypoglycaemic agents and insulin is only occasionally required.

IMPAIRED LUNG FUNCTION. Although lung damage is progressive, if acute exacerbations are treated promptly the rate of deterioration can be minimized.

PNEUMOTHORAX. This occurs most commonly in adults but any patient who suddenly becomes more breathless or complains of chest pain should be examined and have a chest X-ray to exclude a pneumothorax.

HAEMOPTYSIS. Transient haemoptysis is common and is usually harmless. If it is severe bronchial artery ligation may be necessary.

NASAL POLYPS AND SINUSITIS. The majority of patients develop nasal polyps and if they cause symptoms they should be removed. Sinusitis is treated with antibiotics and antral wash-outs if necessary.

LIVER DISEASE. A minority of older patients develop cirrhosis progressing to portal hypertension. Wherever possible treatment should be conservative as the mortality of portacaval shunt operations in these patients is very high.

MECONIUM ILEUS AND 'MECONIUM ILEUS EQUIVALENT'. Meconium ileus in neonates should be treated surgically following rehydration. Some adults develop intestinal obstruction from meconium ileus equivalent' and this should be avoided if possible as the operative mortality is high.

REPRODUCTION. Males with cystic fibrosis are usually infertile because the vasa deferentia are abnormal. Pregnancy in women with cystic fibrosis is hazardous because effective postural drainage is difficult to perform in late pregnancy and restriction of diaphragmatic movement may cause respiratory failure.

Prognosis. With vigorous treatment as outlined the majority of affected patients now survive into the third or fourth decades but most die before 40 years of age from respiratory failure resulting from pulmonary sepsis.

Genetic Counselling. For the parents of a child with cystic fibrosis careful explanation of the risks of further pregnancies must be given i.e. that there is a 1 in 4 risk of them having another affected child and a 1 in 2 risk of having a child who is a carrier. The future partner of any patient with cystic fibrosis who plans to marry should be fully informed of the problems presented by the disease.

Chapter 9

RESPIRATORY FAILURE (including Adult Respiratory Distress Syndrome)

Definition. Respiratory failure is usually defined as present when the arterial oxygen tension is less than 8 kPa (60 mm Hg) or the arterial carbon dioxide tension is above 6·6 kPa (50 mm Hg). In clinical practice conditions most often causing respiratory failure are: chronic airways obstruction (chronic bronchitis and emphysema), asthma, depression of consciousness, pulmonary oedema and other exudates, fibrosing lung diseases, neuromuscular diseases.

Classification. Two types of respiratory failure are recognized:
1. HYPOXAEMIA WITHOUT HYPERCAPNIA. Hyperventilation induced by hypoxia results in normal or excessive carbon dioxide excretion leading to normal or low arterial carbon dioxide tensions ($PaCO_2$). This may occur with extensive pneumonias, pulmonary oedema, diffuse interstitial pulmonary fibrosis or loss of lung tissue from other causes.
2. HYPOXAEMIA WITH HYPERCAPNIA (Ventilatory failure). This results from alveolar hypoventilation, usually as a complication of severe airways obstruction with associated insensitivity of the respiratory centres to rises in arterial carbon dioxide tension or from maldistribution of ventilation and perfusion.

It is important to distinguish between these two types of respiratory failure because if oxygen is given freely to patients with ventilatory failure this will remove the stimulus to ventilation from hypoxia and further carbon dioxide retention will occur.

Aetiology and Functional Abnormalities
1. HYPOXAEMIA WITHOUT HYPERCAPNIA
   Ventilation and Perfusion Imbalance. If some alveoli are under-ventilated relative to their perfusion blood leaving them will have a low oxygen tension and a raised carbon dioxide tension (the '*venous admixture effect*'). This will tend to raise the carbon dioxide tension of the mixed arterial blood and stimulate the respiratory centre to increase ventilation. Increase in ventilation of alveoli already well-ventilated will compensate by excreting excess carbon dioxide because of the linear shape of the carbon dioxide dissociation curve for whole blood but because of the shape of the oxygen dissociation curve for haemoglobin these alveoli will not be able to compensate for the tendency to hypoxia which results from other under ventilated alveoli (*see Fig.* 9). If hyperventilation reduces the carbon dioxide tension below normal levels a compensatory

respiratory alkalosis will develop. This is then corrected by renal excretion of bicarbonate ions. Causes of respiratory failure where ventilation and perfusion imbalance is an important factor include asthma, pneumonia, pulmonary fibrosis, pulmonary oedema and pulmonary collapse. It may also contribute to the hypoxaemia of chronic bronchitis and emphysema.

Impaired Gas Transfer. Thickening of the alveolar capillary membrane is rarely, if ever, of sufficient degree to impair exchange of carbon dioxide and oxygen. However ventilation–perfusion imbalance i.e. mismatching of the distribution of ventilation and perfusion commonly occurs in diseases associated with diffuse pulmonary fibrosis such as the pneumoconioses and fibrosing alveolitis. This mismatching will result in hypoxia without hypercapnia until the disease is very advanced when the remaining well-perfused and ventilated alveoli can no longer compensate for poorly ventilated alveoli and hypercapnia will also develop.

2. HYPOXIA WITH HYPERCAPNIA 'VENTILATORY FAILURE'

Alveolar Hypoventilation. The arterial carbon dioxide tension will rise if there is generalized alveolar hypoventilation. As there is a reciprocal relationship between the partial pressure of carbon dioxide and oxygen in the blood and alveolar air (the nitrogen content remaining fairly constant over short periods), the arterial carbon dioxide tension cannot rise above 12 kPa (90 mm Hg) while the patient is *breathing air* without the arterial oxygen tension falling to lethal levels. Ventilatory failure with carbon dioxide retention is common with chronic airways obstruction from chronic bronchitis but patients with emphysema develop hypercapnic respiratory failure only with very advanced disease. The tendency to develop carbon dioxide retention in most of these patients is associated with a loss of sensitivity of the respiratory centres to carbon dioxide. This is of unknown cause. Ventilation–perfusion imbalance also plays a part in respiratory failure developing in chronic bronchitis and emphysema.

Ventilatory failure is common with depression of consciousness, especially from drug overdoses. Other causes include neurological diseases affecting the brain, spinal cord, intercostal nerves, neuromuscular junctions and respiratory muscles.

Clinical Features. Many breathless patients have normal blood gas tensions while others may have severe hypoxaemia and hypercapnia without breathlessness, this is especially true of patients with chronic bronchitis or those suffering from drug overdoses.

The clinical features of hypoxaemia and hypercapnia are not unique to those conditions.

HYPOXAEMIA. Causes impairment of *cerebral function* presenting as restlessness, agitation and confusion. *Cardiac.* Effects include increased output and heart rate. Chronic hypoxaemia leads to pulmonary hypertension and cor pulmonale and severe hypoxaemia may cause cardiac dysrhythmias, renal failure and hepatic necrosis. Tissue cellular damage does not begin to appear until the arterial oxygen tension falls to about 2·5 kPa (20 mm Hg). With severe hypoxaemia anaerobic tissue metabolism may lead to a lactic acidosis and metabolic acidosis.

HYPERCAPNIA. *Cerebral symptoms* include headache (from cerebral vasodilatation), confusion, drowsiness, coarse muscle twitching and coma. The *circulatory effects* include generalized vasodilatation with warm peripheries, sweating and a wide pulse pressure. Carbon dioxide retention causes a respiratory acidosis and renal compensation occurs by excretion of hydrogen ions and reabsorption of bicarbonate ions. The associated sodium retention and the effects of carbon dioxide on the kidney may cause fluid retention resulting in peripheral oedema without true cardiac failure.

Diagnosis. Because central cyanosis is a late sign of hypoxaemia and the clinical signs of both hypoxaemia and hypercapnia are not specific the diagnosis rests essentially on blood gas analysis and when interpreting the results it is essential to know what concentration of oxygen the patient was breathing at the time the blood sample was taken.

Differential Diagnosis

1. COMA. Carbon dioxide narcosis must be distinguished from other causes of coma, by physical examination, investigations and where possible by history.
2. CYANOTIC HEART DISEASE. This is recognized by the presence of cardiac abnormalities including murmurs. Administration of 35 per cent oxygen abolishes respiratory cyanosis within 3 or 4 minutes while in cyanotic heart disease persistent cyanosis is present due to right-to-left cardiac shunts.
3. SEVERE HAEMORRHAGE. May cause cerebral hypoxaemia but the history, examination and the haemoglobin level will differentiate this from respiratory failure.
4. MENTAL ILLNESS. Occasionally severe respiratory failure with or without hypercapnia may be mistaken for agitation, anxiety and restlessness due to mental illness, especially in the elderly.

Principles of Treatment

1. RECOGNITION OF PRECIPITATING FACTORS
   a. *Injudicious oxygen therapy* may cause alveolar hypoventilation due to loss of the hypoxic drive to respiration in patients with hypercapnia.

    b. Mechanical limitation of respiratory movement following surgery or injury to the abdomen or chest, the presence of gross ascites, as well as neuromuscular defects affecting the chest and abdomen may cause alveolar hypoventilation.

    c. Ventilation–perfusion abnormalities may be exaggerated by pneumonia, large pleural effusions or spontaneous pneumothorax.

2. RELIEF OF VENTILATORY OBSTRUCTION. Treatment aims to reduce mucosal swelling and inflammation and to reduce bronchial secretions and constriction of bronchial smooth muscle.

    The following measures are used:

    a. Physiotherapy to aid coughing and removal of secretions, it also serves to waken drowsy patients with carbon dioxide retention.

    b. Rehydration may reduce sputum viscosity. Although this is seldom a problem with chronic bronchitis it can be very helpful in severe asthma.

    c. Bronchial toilet by suction, bronchoscopy or bronchial lavage may remove tenacious sputum.

    d. Bronchodilator drugs by intravenous infusion or by inhalation should be given to relieve airways obstruction.

    e. Antibiotic therapy for control of bacterial infection.

    f. Avoid sedation: opiates, barbiturates or tranquillizers may precipitate or exaggerate respiratory depression and should be withheld unless the patient is already being artificially ventilated.

    g. Respiratory stimulants: Nikethamide, 3–5 ml of 25 per cent solution by i.v. injection can be given at intervals to arouse the patient for physiotherapy and coughing. Doxapram may be given by i.v. infusion at a rate of 1–2 mg per min but cautious observation for excessive CNS and cardiac stimulation is essential.

3. RELIEF OF HYPOXIA
Cautions

    a. Avoid inducing hypoventilation in patients with poor respiratory drive by excessive administration of oxygen.

    b. The dangers of oxygen toxicity in high concentration must be recognized.

METHODS OF ADMINISTRATION. The underlying principle in treating respiratory failure is to raise the arterial oxygen tension to between 7 and 10 kPa (50–85 mm Hg).

    1. *Hypoxaemia due to Arteriovenous Admixture* ('Shunt'). Caused by pneumonia or severe pulmonary fibrosis without airways obstruction. High concentrations of oxygen (40–60 per cent) may be given without inducing carbon dioxide retention. Suitable equipment includes Pneumo Mask, MC Mask and Nasal Catheters.

    2. *Hypoxaemia with Hypercapnia.* Prior measurement of arterial carbon dioxide tension is invaluable. If there is already carbon dioxide retention treatment should begin with an inspired oxygen

concentration of 24 per cent and only if this causes no further increase in arterial carbon dioxide tension should higher oxygen concentrations of 28 or 35 per cent be used. Suitable masks for this purpose are the Venti Mask series giving 24, 28 and 35 per cent inspired oxygen concentrations.

Other methods of oxygen administration:

1. *Nasal Catheters.* May be used in patients who will not tolerate a mask. Good control of inspired concentration is difficult with this method and it is unsuitable where carbon dioxide retention is a danger.

2. *Head Tent.* This may be useful for the latter group. These, too, work on the Venturi principle to provide controlled oxygen therapy. Conventional oxygen tents which give uncontrolled oxygen concentrations are probably only now needed for treating childhood illness and are dangerous if hypercapnia is a hazard.

DOMICILIARY OXYGEN. Some patients with severe chronic respiratory failure may benefit from a home oxygen supply enabling them to move more freely and cope with essential tasks such as washing, dressing and moving about. Small portable oxygen kits, sufficient for 10–15 minutes exertion, are available which can be refilled from a larger cylinder delivered to the house.

LONG-TERM OXYGEN THERAPY. Continuous administration of low concentrations of oxygen for 14–16 hours each day may possibly bring about sustained reduction in pulmonary arterial pressure. This is under investigation.

HAZARDS OF OXYGEN THERAPY

1. *Hypoventilation* is the main risk in patients with impaired carbon dioxide sensitivity who rely upon the hypoxic drive to respiration.

2. *Withdrawal of Oxygen.* Because the body stores may contain up to 17 litres of carbon dioxide but there are no tissue stores for oxygen, sudden withdrawal of oxygen once oxygen enrichment has begun may lead to a catastrophic fall in the alveolar oxygen tension resulting in profound hypoxaemia. Oxygen therapy once begun, must be continued without interruption until ventilation has improved.

3. *Retrolental Fibroplasia.* If high inspired concentrations of oxygen above about 18 kPa (150 mm Hg) are maintained in neonates for long period retrolental fibroplasia may develop.

4. *Pulmonary Oxygen Toxicity.* Prolonged inhalation of high concentrations of oxygen (above 60 per cent) will cause alveolar capillary proliferation, intra-alveolar haemorrhages and exudates, fibroblast proliferation and desquamation of alveolar lining cells, leading to gross disturbance of gas exchange. In addition, removal

of nitrogen from the alveoli may lead to absorption collapse of alveoli with atelectasis.

OTHER MEASURES. Diuretics may reduce fluid retention and are also valuable in heart failure complicating respiratory failure. Digoxin should be used with great caution because when used with patients in sinus rhythm there is no simple clinical guide to the presence of digoxin toxicity. Corticosteroids (i.v. hydrocortisone) may be helpful.

ARTIFICIAL VENTILATION. Artificial ventilation should not be started unless the underlying disease is likely to be reversible or controllable within the foreseeable future. Ventilation through an endotracheal tube alone is possible for 3–7 days but for longer periods a tracheostomy is necessary.

Indications Include:

1. Increasing respiratory rate and tachycardia.
2. Development of hypotension.
3. The patient is becoming exhausted.
4. Anxiety and restlessness, progressing to drowsiness and confusion.
5. Progressive deterioration in arterial blood gas tensions.

Artificial ventilation allows:

1. Adequate control of ventilation.
2. Relief of hypoxia with slow controlled reduction of hypercapnia, thus preventing cerebral effects from sudden changes in arterial carbon dioxide tension.
3. Relief of the workload of breathing.
4. Improved bronchial toilet.

As with other forms of oxygen therapy the aim should be to maintain arterial oxygen tensions as close to normal as possible, in the range of 9–12 kPa (65–100 mm Hg).

ADULT RESPIRATORY DISTRESS SYNDROME (ARDS)

Shock lung, wet lung, congestive atelectasis.

Introduction. This form of progressive respiratory failure was first encountered with non-thoracic war injuries but other recognized causes include road traffic and other civilian accidents, fat and amniotic fluid embolism, severe septicaemia, acute viral pneumonia, blast injuries and cardiopulmonary bypass.

Clinical Features. These include tachypnoea, a low arterial oxygen tension in spite of high inspired oxygen concentration and diffuse patchy shadows on chest X-ray. There is a latent period between the injury and the onset of symptoms. As the hypoxia worsens tachypnoea and tachycardia develop accompanied by signs of cerebral anoxia. Examination of the chest usually reveals few abnormal signs.

Pathology. There is interstitial and intra-alveolar oedema, perivascular haemorrhage with bleeding into alveoli and thrombo-emboli in pulmonary vessels. Fibrin or fibrinogen hyaline membranes line affected alveoli and fibroblast proliferation leads to widespread fibrosis.

Pathogenesis. Two main mechanisms are thought to be involved:
1. Spasm of small pulmonary veins.
2. Increased permeability of pulmonary capillaries.

Physiological Disturbances. Lung compliance is reduced and the dead space–tidal volume ratio is increased. There is gross widening of the alveolar–arterial oxygen tension gradient due to 'shunts' caused by non-ventilated and poorly ventilated alveoli.

> CHEST X-RAY. This may appear normal following fat or amniotic fluid embolism but subsequently extensive 'fluffy' shadowing develops and may be followed by complete 'white out' of the lung fields.

Treatment. Avoid overtransfusion and when large volumes of stored blood are used it must be carefully filtered. Oxygen enrichment of inspired gases should be controlled to give the lowest inspired oxygen concentration that will maintain adequate arterial oxygen tensions. Most patients require mechanical ventilation. Great benefit is claimed for the use of positive end-expiratory pressures during artificial ventilation. High doses of cortico-steroids (methylprednisolone 30 mg per kg) have been advocated for treatment in the first 48 hours.

Prognosis. This depends upon the individual mechanism leading to the development of ARDS. Complete recovery with normal lung function is possible but most survivors show a persistent restrictive ventilatory defect.

Chapter 10

BRONCHIAL ASTHMA

Definition. Bronchial asthma is characterized by breathlessness and wheezing caused by generalized narrowing of intrapulmonary airways which varies in severity spontaneously or as a result of treatment. Symptoms may be persistent but are usually recurrent and paroxysmal.

Epidemiology. Studies from various countries have shown a similar prevalence for asthma, between 0·5 and 2·0 per cent of the population of all ages being affected, but it is much commoner in some isolated communities. Asthma may begin at any age but between 5 and 10 per cent of all children wheeze before the age of 10 years and in this group boys are affected twice as often as girls. Later in life the incidence of asthma is higher in women than men.

Pathology. The changes recognized from post-mortem studies include hypertrophy and hyperplasia of bronchial smooth muscle, thickening of the epithelial basement membrane of the airways, eosinophilic infiltration of the bronchial wall, hypertrophy of bronchial mucous glands, increased numbers of goblet cells, and plugging of bronchi and bronchioles with viscid mucus-containing eosinophils and respiratory epithelial cells (*Fig.* 22). The lungs of patients dying from asthma usually show overinflation with widespread mucous plugs in the airways.

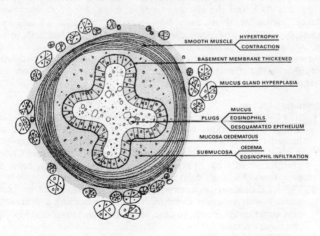

Fig. 22. Diagram of the changes in the bronchial wall in asthma.

Aetiology and Pathogenesis. The pathological changes recognized as characteristic of asthma may seemingly result from a number of different pathogenic mechanisms. Previous subdivision of patients with asthma into polar groups labelled 'extrinsic' and 'intrinsic' seems an oversimplification as patients of either group may be susceptible to the same aggravating factors and may respond to similar treatment.

Extrinsic asthma refers to those patients in whom exacerbations of asthma seem to be precipitated by hypersensitivity to antigenic materials including pollens, feathers, animal fur, house dust and the house dust mite, *Dermatophagoides pteronyssinus,* and fungal spores. Less often foods including milk, eggs, fish, chocolate and alcoholic drinks may precipitate episodes of wheezing. Most patients with this type of asthma are atopic, that is, in addition to positive immediate hypersensitivity (Gell and Coombs Type I) to skin prick tests with extracts of common allergens they have a high incidence of seasonal rhinitis and flexural eczema. Extrinsic asthma usually begins early in life.

In *intrinsic asthma* recognizable allergic features are absent and the age of onset is later. Most accounts of the pathogenesis of asthma emphasize the role played by bronchial smooth muscle, not only because of the striking hypertrophy demonstrated histologically but also because of the improvements in airflow obtained by the use of sympathomimetic and theophylline compounds. The mechanisms controlling airway calibre in asthma are probably the result of the interaction of a number of factors including a balance between neural impulses from both the parasympathetic (vagal, cholinergic) and sympathetic (beta and alpha adrenergic) nervous impulses, and the effects of one or more of the following possible chemical mediators: histamine, slow reacting substance of anaphylaxis (SRSA), lysosomes, and prostaglandins released from *Mast* cells or other sites. A minority of patients with asthma may develop symptoms from a single cause such as allergy to pollens or exercise but most patients are susceptible to the effects of more than one mechanism. Only parts of the causal pathways are understood (*Fig.* 23).

Precipitating Factors

1. HYPERSENSITIVITY MECHANISMS. Most patients with 'allergic' asthma develop symptoms as a result of Type I (Gell and Coombs) immediate reagin-(IgE antibody) mediated hypersensitivity but in a small proportion of these patients Type III (Gell and Coombs) precipitin-mediated hypersensitivity mechanisms may cause later symptoms of asthma delayed in onset by 8–12 hours.

2. EXERCISE. Many patients with asthma, especially children, become wheezy with vigorous exercise. Typically wheezing and breathlessness come on after a short time, less often symptoms develop during sustained exertion.

3. INFECTION. Common respiratory infections frequently precipitate

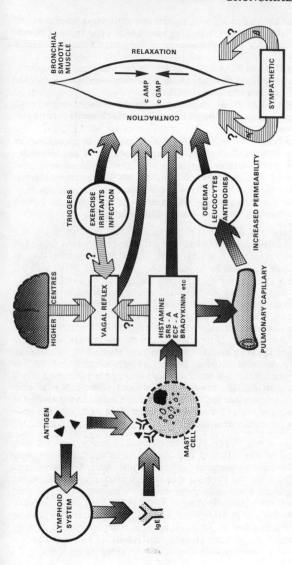

Fig. 23. Diagram of some of the mechanisms which may cause air-ways obstruction in asthma. SRS–A, slow reacting substance of anaphylaxis. ECF–A, eosinophil chemotactic factor of anaphy-laxis. cAMP, cyclic 3'5' adenosine monophosphate. cGMP, cyclic 3'5' guanosine monophosphate.

episodes of asthma at all ages. In children rhinovirus infections are especially likely to cause wheezing but in adults the types of micro-organisms causing exacerbations of asthma have been less clearly defined.

4. NON-SPECIFIC IRRITANTS. Changes in temperature, atmospheric conditions, exposure to cigarette smoke and non-antigenic dusts are all potential causes of asthma attacks.

5. EMOTIONAL FACTORS. Acute episodes are often associated with psychological upset but the relationship of psychogenic factors and asthma is complex.

6. DRUGS. Allergic (Type I) reactions to drugs, such as penicillin may precipitate asthma. Salicylates and other analgesics are especially likely to provoke asthma in patients with the combination of late-onset asthma and nasal polyps through non-allergic mechanisms. Propranolol and other beta-sympathomimetic antagonists may increase or precipitate airways obstruction in patients with asthma at all ages, through beta-sympathetic blockade.

Physiological Changes in Asthma. The cardinal feature is airways obstruction which may not be detectable between attacks, but is often present in the absence of symptoms or abnormal signs. Simple measurements such as PEFR or FEV_1 and FVC will be impaired and the ratio of FEV_1 to FVC will be reduced. During acute episodes the lungs may be overinflated so that TLC, FRC and RV may be increased above predicted levels and in many instances improvement is accompanied by a reduction in these lung volumes. Gas transfer is usually well preserved in asthma except in severe exacerbations, in contrast to emphysema, allowing the differentiation to be made between these two conditions. Blood gas measurements will usually give normal results between attacks but often patients may be significantly hypoxic without apparent distress. Despite airways obstruction there is usually alveolar overventilation which causes hypocapnia but during severe exacerbations carbon dioxide retention may occur when this overventilation no longer compensates for the effects of the many underventilated alveoli. This is a grave sign. Chronic respiratory failure and cor pulmonale are rarely seen in patients with asthma.

Chest X-ray. The chest X-ray is often normal in many patients with asthma but signs of overinflation such as low flat diaphragms are commonly present even in remission and bronchial wall thickening and prominence of the hilar and perihilar shadows are often present on routine chest X-rays. Patients with pulmonary eosinophilia may show transient shadows during exacerbations leading to nodular shadows and parallel or ring and band shadows with established damage. Bronchography will show the characteristic dilatation of proximal bronchi with established damage from allergic bronchopulmonary aspergillosis. Rarely in an acute episode a pneumothorax or a pneumomediastinum may be detected on X-ray.

Clinical Features of Asthma. In episodic asthma, between attacks there may be no abnormal signs. Patients with marked airways obstruction may present without complaints but usually in the presence of airways obstruction there is breathlessness, wheezing and cough productive of variable quantities of mucoid sputum which may be green if eosinophils are present in excess. Curschmann's spirals consist of viscid plugs of mucus which are coughed up. Symptoms are especially likely to occur at night or in the early hours of the morning. There is commonly marked diurnal variation with most severe airways obstruction in the mornings.

Physical Examination. In exacerbations the respiratory rate is usually raised and the accessory muscles of respiration are used. Visible signs indicating airways obstruction include recession of the intercostal spaces and supraclavicular fossae, shortening of the space from the suprasternal notch to the thyroid cartilage, downward 'tug' of the thyroid cartilage on inspiration, engorgement of the jugular veins on expiration and pulsus paradoxus. The chest may appear fixed and overinflated and the areas of cardiac and liver dullness may be reduced. Inspiratory and expiratory rhonchi will be audible and expiration is prolonged, with very severe airways obstruction the breath sounds may become almost inaudible – beware *the quiet chest*. There may be severe hypoxia without cyanosis, because this is an unreliable sign due to variations in skin colour, lighting and observer error.

Patterns of Asthma

CHILDHOOD ASTHMA. Wheeziness is common in infancy with minor respiratory tract infections but is also present in acute bronchiolitis. Wheezing not associated with asthma clears as lung growth continues. Factors which indicate that persistent asthma is likely to occur include a family history of asthma, recurrent episodes of wheezing, usually with infections, in the first three years of life and a persistence of wheezing at 10 years of age. About 25 per cent of children with severe asthma and 50 per cent of those with intermittent mild attacks may be symptom free by the age of 15.

ADULT ASTHMA. Asthma may begin at any age but about 90 per cent of males who have asthma have their first episodes before the age of 35 years but the onset of symptoms after this age occurs in about a quarter of women with asthma.

EPISODIC ASTHMA. Many patients with a background of good health may have intermittent acute episodes of asthma precipitated by respiratory infections, increase in the pollen count, the interplay of emotional factors or sudden exposure to irritants such as smog or cigarette smoke and with vigorous exercise or laughing.

CHRONIC ASTHMA. Many adults and some children may have chronic wheezing and breathlessness without good remissions. Superimposed on this persistent airways obstruction acute exacerbations may occur due to the same factors previously mentioned.

STATUS ASTHMATICUS. There is no universally accepted definition of this condition. It is commonly used to refer to patients who have had severe wheezing and breathlessness lasting more than 24 hours but life-threatening episodes may be of much shorter duration. Patients may have central cyanosis and be too breathless to walk about or speak. In very severe episodes restlessness and disturbance of consciousness may develop. Other important signs are a pulse rate greater than 100 per minute, pulsus paradoxus and very quiet breath sounds on auscultation.

Differential Diagnosis

1. ACUTE BRONCHITIS. This is common in children and adults. Differentiation from episodic asthma is helped by a history of recurrent episodes, family history of asthma, eczema or hay fever and the presence of a blood or sputum eosinophilia.

2. CHRONIC BRONCHITIS. Confusion may occur in adult patients with wheezing and breathlessness. The coexistence of asthma and chronic bronchitis is not uncommon and in all such patients search for blood and sputum eosinophilia. Test for reversibility of airways obstruction with bronchodilators and if necessary corticosteroids (see Chapter 18).

3. PULMONARY OEDEMA. Severe breathlessness and wheezing may occur with acute pulmonary oedema and especially in elderly patients may mimic PND; careful examination and investigation may be necessary to differentiate between 'cardiac asthma' and bronchial asthma. A careful history is usually invaluable in making this distinction.

4. PULMONARY EMBOLISM. Sudden severe breathlessness due to acute massive pulmonary embolus may rarely present with wheezing. Signs of right heart failure will dominate the clinical picture.

Investigations

1. BLOOD. An absolute eosinophil count may be helpful, counts above $0.5 \times 10^9/l$ in the absence of parasitic infestation support a clinical diagnosis of asthma. Counts in excess of $1.0 \times 10^9/l$ are common with pulmonary eosinophilia from any cause.

2. SPUTUM. The presence of eosinophils is helpful in diagnosis and Charcot—Leyden crystals and Curschman's spirals consisting of inspissated mucus and shed epithelial cells are commonly present in the sputum in asthma.

3. PULMONARY FUNCTION TESTS. Simple measurements of air flow including PEFR, FEV_1, FVC before and after inhalation of a bronchodilator aerosol are helpful. An increase of more than 20 per

cent in PEFR or FEV_1 are strongly suggestive of asthma but in severe episodes and with persistent asthma there may be no change after a bronchodilator. More complex measurements of lung function are only necessary in a minority of patients.

4. CHEST X-RAY. This may be normal in many patients but over-inflation is often detectable and occasionally a pneumothorax, pneumomediastinum or pulmonary infiltrates may be present in addition to signs of bronchial wall thickening.

5. TESTS FOR HYPERSENSITIVITY. Skin prick tests with prepared solutions of antigenic material will identify those patients who are atopic, but only in a minority of patients will this lead to important therapeutic measures. Inhalation challenge tests may very occasionally be indicated especially where occupational asthma is suspected. These must be done in hospital under carefully controlled conditions because severe delayed asthmatic reactions often occur.

Treatment

1. PREVENTIVE MEASURES. Commonly in children and occasionally in adults careful attention to the avoidance of potential antigens may be very helpful in management. Reduction in the house dust mite population by daily airing the bed clothing, vacuum cleaning of mattresses and furnishings and substitution of synthetic fibres for feathers and wool may be helpful. Occasionally the removal of domestic animals may lead to improvement but care should be taken to confirm any indications from skin tests by clinical observations. Many a cat has been slain in vain! Seasonal asthma whether due to spring pollens or autumn moulds can be helped by sensible behaviour, avoiding over exposure to causative agents. *Desensitization* has been shown to be effective with aqueous extracts of grass pollens but the effectiveness of other extracts, except perhaps for house dust mite, is disappointing. The ideal patient for desensitization is one with a single positive skin reaction to pollens.

2. BRONCHODILATORS. For episodic asthma treatment with bronchodilators alone may be successful. Where possible these drugs should be given by aerosol as this route of administration results in longer duration of effect with fewer systemic side effects.

   Aerosols. Pressurized aerosols of beta-adrenergic sympathomimetic compounds are very valuable. The newer relatively selective drugs including salbutamol (Ventolin), terbutaline (Bricanyl), rimiterol (Pulmadil) and fenoterol (Berotec) are safer than isoprenaline as they are less cardiotoxic and are longer lasting. When they are prescribed it is necessary to check that the patient has mastered the technique of using such aerosols and clear instructions should be given of a maximum number of inhalations which should not be exceeded without seeking medical advice.

Oral Bronchodilator Drugs. A wide variety of combination compounds is available most of which contain suboptimal doses of active agents. For childhood asthma simple ephedrine or theophylline tablets may be helpful and those containing barbiturates should be avoided. There are theoretical grounds for believing the theophylline compounds have a different mode of action from the sympathomimetic agents and although they may cause nausea and gastrointestinal upset they do not give rise to muscle tremor and tachycardia, which are common with the sympathomimetic drugs. It may be useful to combine an oral theophylline bronchodilator with an aerosol of a sympathomimetic compound. In general it is best to avoid giving oral preparations of the sympathomimetic type.

Disodium Cromoglycate (DSCG; Intal). This is a valuable prophylactic agent presently available for inhalation in powder form from a capsule using a spinhaler. It is effective in a minority of patients (perhaps 30–40 per cent) with all types of asthma and should always be given a proper trial before it is discarded. The compound preparation which contains isoprenaline should not be used as it confuses assessment. For Intal to be effective airway calibre should be improved by other means so that Intal can be distributed throughout the bronchial tree. The conventional dose of one capsule four times daily in combination with bronchodilator treatment and objective assessment over a period of 4–6 weeks is desirable, but some patients who fail to respond to this dose may improve with a larger dose. Patients in whom exercise-induced asthma is a problem and those where specific allergic factors are recognized often find that prophylactic use of an additional capsule of Intal shortly before exposure may be helpful.

Corticosteroid Aerosols. Two highly active topical corticosteroid preparations with low glucocorticoid activity are available, beclomethasone dipropionate (Becotide) and betamethasone 17-valerate (Bextasol). There is little to choose between them. These should be given in the recommended dose of 2 puffs four times daily. These compounds can be used in combination with bronchodilators to control troublesome episodic or mild persistent asthma and in addition have been shown to have important 'steroid-sparing' effects allowing a previous dose of oral corticosteroid to be at least halved in most cases. Oropharyngeal candidiasis occurs in about 10 per cent of patients but the incidence is much higher when larger doses are used. There have been no reports of candidiasis distal to the larynx but the long-term effects of topical application of steroids to the respiratory mucosa has not yet been assessed. *It is important* that patients on steroid aerosols should understand that these have a different mode of action from bronchodilators, that they must not be discontinued suddenly and that they will be ineffective if airways obstruction becomes severe.

Oral Steroid Therapy. There are no proven advantages to the new synthetic corticosteroids compared with prednisone or prednisolone in standard preparation or enteric-coated where gastrointestinal symptoms are a problem.

a. *Short-course Treatment:* For any acute exacerbation of asthma which fails to respond to intensive bronchodilator treatment early use of corticosteroids is invaluable. Prednisolone 30 mg daily in divided doses is effective in all but a minority of patients and this dose should be continued unchanged until maximum improvement has occurred as recorded by frequent measurements of PEFR, usually within 5–7 days. Once adequate bronchodilatation has been achieved treatment with a steroid aerosol should be started during the continuation phase of the oral treatment. Thereafter the oral dose may be reduced rapidly to zero over a further 5–7 days without risk of persistent hypothalamo-pituitary-adrenal suppresion, provided that the patient has not had previous maintenance treatment with corticosteroids.

b. *Corticosteroid Diagnostic Test:* In patients with persistent airflow obstruction which is suspected to be due to asthma a similar course of prednisolone 30 mg daily should be tried with measurements of PEFR. If no improvement in PEFR occurs within 10–14 days corticosteroids should be discontinued. Where improvement occurs a corticosteroid aerosol may be substituted during the period of oral treatment as described above.

c. *Long-term Treatment:* In a minority of patients with persistent asthma control by bronchodilators and steroid aerosols alone may be ineffective. Other patients may present for treatment who have already been started on systemic corticosteroids. Here the aim should be to achieve optimal control of asthma with the minimum total dose of corticosteroids. In all patients an attempt should be made to continue with the recommended dose of a steroid aerosol and the daily dose of oral prednisolone should be adjusted to the minimum which maintains satisfactory symptomatic and objective control. For this purpose combination treatment with 5-mg and 1-mg tablets may be necessary. Clearly careful instruction of the patient is required.

Alternate-day Corticosteroids: The side effects of corticosteroid treatment can be reduced if these drugs are given on alternate days. Thus prednisolone 20 mg on alternate days will give similar control with less adrenal suppression etc. as prednisolone 10 mg daily. Where alternate-day treatment is given from the onset it is usually successful but once a patient has been on daily steroid treatment attempts to change to an alternate-day regimen are usually unsuccessful.

SIDE EFFECTS. The majority of patients will be satisfactorily controlled with a daily dose of 7·5 mg prednisolone or less. Side effects are not a problem. Above this level Cushingoid features appear but weight gain can be controlled by dietary restriction. Regular checks for glucose intolerance and gastrointestinal symptoms should always be made but fortunately osteoporosis with skeletal problems is uncommon in patients with asthma. Where patients require more than 10 mg of prednisolone daily for control of asthma optimal management of symptoms with minimum side effects may be achieved by a change to an alternate-day regimen giving double that daily dose on alternate days.

ANTIBIOTICS. It is unlikely that bacterial infections are a major cause of exacerbations of asthma but the majority of patients in whom infections seems to be an important precipitant find that prompt treatment with a broad-spectrum antibiotic is helpful. Ampicillin, amoxycillin, co-trimoxazole or tetracycline for 5–7 days in conventional doses is usually adequate.

Treatment of the Severe Attack. When a severe episode of asthma develops, especially where it persists without relief for more than 24 hours there is always the risk of death from exhaustion and respiratory failure. Danger signs are disturbance of consciousness, difficulty with speech because of breathlessness, a heart rate of 100/min or more, pulsus paradoxus and PEFR of 60 l/min or less. Many patients will be cyanosed but severe hypoxaemia may be present without cyanosis.

Hypoxia must be relieved by humidified oxygen as soon as possible and dehydration resulting from hyperventilation and inadequate fluid intake should be relieved by oral fluids if possible otherwise an i.v. infusion of normal saline should be given. Arterial blood gas tensions and hydrogen ion content should be measured; any degree of hypercapnia is a dangerous finding.

Sedatives must not be given. Bronchodilator treatment may be given with aminophylline or salbutamol (Ventolin) by slow i.v. infusion. Subcutaneous adrenaline or terbutaline (Bricanyl) are other suitable parenteral bronchodilators. In addition salbutamol may be given by inhalation with intermittent positive-pressure breathing or a nebulizer driven by compressed air. The heart rate must be carefully watched to ensure that the bronchodilators are not causing undue tachycardia and in very severe cases an ECG monitor should be used.

The majority of patients will require corticosteroids. In the moderately ill patient who is able to drink, prednisolone may be given by mouth starting with a dose of 40–60 mg daily. In most cases it is customary to begin corticosteroid treatment with i.v. hydrocortisone in doses of the order of 4 mg/kg bodyweight at 4–6-hourly intervals, changing to oral prednisolone after 24–48 hours. Where large doses of hydrocortisone are used potassium supplements must be given to replace urinary losses.

Artificial ventilation by intermittant positive-pressure ventilation (IPPV) is indicated for patients who present with severe clouding of consciousness or who are moribund. Other indications for IPPV after the start of treatment are exhaustion and progressive deterioration in arterial blood gas tensions, especially a rising pCO_2, in spite of intensive treatment. The details of the management of IPPV for severe asthma are beyond the scope of this book, suffice it to say that it is advisable to call on the services of an anaesthetist or physician with special experience of this difficult technique. Patients with severe episodes of asthma are generally given a course of a broad-spectrum antibiotic although few such episodes have been proved to be due to bacterial infection. It is rarely necessary to give i.v. sodium bicarbonate to correct severe acidosis and the need for bronchial lavage to remove viscid mucus has a few enthusiastic advocates although most centres seem to find it is rarely indicated.

Chapter 11

ACUTE RESPIRATORY TRACT INFECTIONS

Common Cold; Pharyngitis; Tracheobronchitis; Bronchiolitis; Influenza; Pneumonia (*see* Chapter 12).

Respiratory tract infections, the commonest affliction of mankind, are most often caused by viruses. Most respiratory viruses can cause a range of clinical syndromes from the common cold to pneumonia; although primary viral pneumonia is rare it is common for secondary bacterial pneumonia to follow in the wake of a respiratory virus infection. Because of the continuity of the mucosa of the respiratory tract precise localization of a virus infection to one part of the tracheobronchial tube is unlikely to be common but some viruses are usually associated with symptoms suggestive of dominant effects on the upper or lower respiratory tract (*Table* 3).

Table 3. Common respiratory pathogens and related syndromes

Infective Agents	Colds	'Influenza' and febrile	Croup	Bron-chitis	Bronchi-olitis	Pneumonia (children under 5 years)
Influenza A, B	+	++	+	+	−	+
Parainfluenza 1−4	+	+	++	+	+	+
Respiratory syncytial virus	+	+	+	+	++	+
Adenovirus	+	+	+	+	−	+
Picornavirus (rhinoviruses and some enteroviruses	++	+	−	++	−	−

++ = commonly associated.
 + = less often associated.
 − = rarely associated.

COMMON COLD

Aetiology and Pathology. The common cold is most often caused by rhinoviruses (*Table* 3). The incubation period is 2−3 days for rhinoviruses and 4 days for respiratory syncytial virus and para-influenza viruses. Neutralizing antibodies against any one of over 100 strains of rhinoviruses can be found in two-thirds of adults and the reservoir of infection is probably maintained by a continuous succession of infecting viruses within any population. Individuals suffer between 2 and 10 viral respiratory infections in a year. Susceptibility is highest in pre-school children and decreases with age.

Virus infection causes oedema and shedding of the columnar respiratory epithelium by 3 days from the onset and regeneration takes a further 10–14 days.

Clinical Features. Rhinorrhoea, nasal obstruction, conjunctivitis and sore throat may be accompanied by a fever of 38–39°C. Secondary extension of infection beyond the nasopharynx with bacteria, particularly pneumococci and *H. influenzae,* commonly occurs leading to sinusitis, otitis media, bronchitis or pneumonia.

Treatment. Specific antiviral agents are not available for general use in respiratory viral infections. Children should be kept in a warm atmosphere and in adults absence from work is usually only necessary if constitutional symptoms are marked. For uncomplicated colds specific treatment is not indicated. Vasoconstrictors may delay healing and should only be used for severe nasal or Eustachian tube obstruction. Antibiotics should be restricted to patients at special risk such as those with chronic lung or cardiac disease. Amoxycillin 250 mg 8-hourly or oxytetracycline 250 mg 6-6-hourly for 5–7 days are usually effective.

ACUTE PHARYNGITIS

Viral infections are the usual cause but streptococci are responsible for some cases. Effects include pharyngeal mucosal inflammation, enlargement of the tonsils and adenoids with yellowish exudates on the tonsils and tender enlargement of the cervical lymph glands. Sore throat and cough are the dominant symptoms but coryzal symptoms are often absent. Fever, malaise and hoarseness may occur.

Treatment. With warmth and adequate fluids, gargling with soluble aspirin may help relieve local discomfort. Penicillin is the drug of choice for streptococcal infections, otherwise tetracycline or erythromycin should be given for secondary bacterial infection.

ACUTE LARYNGOTRACHEOBRONCHITIS (Croup)

In infancy, the commonest cause is infection with para-influenza viruses 1 and 2 or respiratory syncytial virus, but in older children influenza and adenoviruses are the usual causes. Superinfection with haemolytic streptococci and staphylococci sometimes occurs.

Clinical Features. Croup in small children is a serious illness with cough, dyspnoea, *inspiratory stridor* and cyanosis. Fever and systemic upset are variable. The onset may be sudden or follow symptoms of a common cold. Severe airways obstruction leads to marked use of the accessory muscles and intercostal recession on inspiration. Respiratory failure with profound cyanosis and death may occur. The risk is greatest in the first two years of life.

Treatment. Warm humid inhalations may help and failure to respond within 24 hours or the appearance of purulent sputum calls for antibiotic treatment with amoxycillin or erythromycin. Tetracyclines should not be given to children and pregnant women to avoid staining developing teeth and bones. Sleeplessness from coughing may be helped by suitable doses of chloral hydrate or an antihistamine such as chlorpheniramine. In several cases admission to hospital for oxygen therapy and early tracheostomy is advisable, here a short course of corticosteroids may reduce mucosal oedema.

ACUTE EPIGLOTTITIS

This is a rare infection usually caused by *H. influenzae* type B, affecting adults and children.

Clinical Features. The onset is rapid with severe sore throat, dysphagia, cough and fever of 38–39°C without hoarseness because the larynx is spared. Stridor, breathlessness and marked constitutional upset are common.

Treatment. Early treatment with antibiotics is of paramount importance, amoxycillin is the drug of choice and cloxacillin may be advisable in addition to prevent staphylococcal superinfection. Intravenous corticosteroids should be given immediately, hydrocortisone hemisuccinate 100–300 mg at 4–6-hour intervals is suitable for children and adults. Tracheostomy may be necessary especially in very young children.

ACUTE BRONCHIOLITIS

This is usually caused by respiratory syncytial virus infection in very young children.

Clinical Features. Severe dyspnoea with short, grunting respirations, severe cyanosis and constitutional symptoms with a fever of 38–40°C. The main sign on auscultation is widespread coarse crackles.

Treatment. Oxygen and humidification will be needed in severe cases, antibiotics are of no value unless superinfection occurs.

ACUTE TRACHEITIS AND BRONCHITIS

Superinfection of the lower respiratory tract with *S. pneumoniae* and *H. influenzae* causing tracheitis and bronchitis is a frequent complication of the common cold, influenza and severe episodes of measles and whooping cough.

Clinical Features. The onset may be insidious with an irritating dry cough and retrosternal soreness or pain with tracheitis. There may be no abnormal signs in the chest but with bronchitis wheezes will be audible and crepitations will indicate involvement of smaller bronchi and bronchioles. The sputum is usually mucopurulent but may occasionally show traces of blood. Systemic upset varies from minimal to a fever of 38–39°C with dyspnoea and cyanosis.

Radiological Features. In the absence of pneumonia and complicating diseases such as chronic bronchitis and emphysema chest X-ray is usually normal.

Treatment. For uncomplicated tracheitis a warm atmosphere and a cough suppressant such as codeine linctus are all that is necessary. For acute bronchitis with purulent sputum early treatment with tetracycline 250–500 mg 6-hourly or amoxycillin 250 mg 8-hourly are advisable for 5 to 7 days. In a severe exacerbation complicating chronic lung or heart disease prompt treatment with penicillin 1 megaunit and streptomycin 0·5 g twice daily for 7 days may be advisable. Where marked airways obstruction occurs oral or i.v. aminophylline or salbutamol will be helpful. Corticosteroids should only be given for severe exacerbations complicating chronic airways obstruction. A dose of 30–60 mg of prednisolone daily should be effective.

INFLUENZA

Three antigenic strains A, B and C are endemic to all countries but epidemics are caused sporadically by A or B viruses and world pandemics of influenza A occur at intervals of 25–30 years. Mutant forms of the viruses are responsible for outbreaks of highly infectious illness. Infection with influenza viruses causes extensive damage to the respiratory mucosa and secondary bacterial invasion particularly by *S. pyogenes* is common.

Clinical Features. The incubation period of 36–48 hours ends with the abrupt onset of fever, malaise, headache and cough. Generalized muscular aches, anorexia and prostration follow. Constitutional symptoms are dominant and respiratory symptoms of sore throat and nasal congestion are not usually marked. The fever of 39–40°C settles in 2–4 days if complications do not follow. Constitutional symptoms subside but a cough with purulent sputum from secondary bacterial invasion may persist. Symptoms of mild depression are common after influenza.

Complications. Bacterial superinfection is common. Rarely, primary influenzal pneumonia may cause profound illness with life-threatening respiratory failure in previously normal individuals. Uncommon complications include encephalitis, myelopathy, polyneuropathy, myositis, organic dementia, pericarditis and cardiac arrhythmias.

Diagnosis. In epidemics a presumptive diagnosis is usually correct but at other times a few cases are confirmed by laboratory methods of virus isolation and rises in serum antibody titres.

Treatment. For uncomplicated influenza bed rest, aspirin and a high fluid intake suffice. Antibiotics should be reserved for those patients with a history of chronic lung or heart disease or otitis media and those in whom complications ensue. Tetracycline 250 mg 6-hourly or amoxycillin 250 mg three times daily for 7 days are suitable. The treatment of staphylococcal pneumonia is described elsewhere (Chapter 12).

PNEUMONIA

Pneumonia is an inflammatory process affecting the alveoli and adjacent airways, most often caused by infection with micro-organisms but sometimes occurring as a result of allergic, physical or chemical injury. The conventional classification into lobar and bronchial pneumonia is less relevant since the decline in incidence of acute pneumococcal lobar pneumonia and the introduction of antibiotics which usually modify the pathological features from an early stage.

Pathology. Inflammation probably begins in the airways and spreads through the alveoli. In classic *lobar pneumonia* caused by *S. pneumoniae,* because of the virulence of the organism this spreads rapidly to involve an entire lobe, though why it should remain so confined is uncertain. In *lobular* or *bronchopneumonia* infection is limited to a patchy distribution around bronchi distributed irregularly through the lung. The inflammatory reaction begins with vasodilatation leading to the outpouring of an exudate containing red cells, leucocytes, macrophages and fibrin formation. With virulent pneumonias, especially if the immune mechanisms are faulty, micro-organisms may enter the blood stream and in extreme cases lead to septicaemia with infection of other organs such as the brain and kidney. Resolution of the pneumonia consists of phagocytosis of organisms and debris by leucocytes and macrophages. The two phases of inflammation and resolution were referred to as red and grey hepatization in lobar pneumonia but this sequence is now usually modified early by antibiotic treatment. In severe pneumonias, especially with staphylococcal infection following influenza, necrosis of lung tissue may lead to abscess formation followed by extensive scarring. Similarly the inflammatory and fibrotic changes of pneumonia can result in bronchiectatic changes of the affected bronchi.

CAUSATIVE ORGANISMS. Most pneumonias are caused by bacteria. Viruses can cause primary pneumonias but it is much more common for secondary bacterial infection to cause pneumonia as a complication of preceding influenza or other respiratory virus infection which has impaired the defences of the lung.

PNEUMONIA IN PREVIOUSLY HEALTHY PEOPLE. The commonest causes are:

Bacteria: S. pneumoniae; S. pyogenes – especially in influenza epidemics; *Klebsiella pneumoniae.*

Mycoplasma: M. pneumoniae – this is the commonest cause of pneumonia in the previously healthy young.

More rare causes:

Chlamydia: psittacosis-ornithosis.

Rickettsia: R. burnetti—Q fever.

*Legionnaires': * probably caused by a bacterium.

*Viral: * True primary viral pneumonia is rare. Influenza viruses. Adenoviruses.

Pneumonia with pre-existing disease:

Common causes:

Bacteria: S. pneumoniae; S. aureus; H. influenzae — especially with chronic bronchitis.

Less common:

Bacteria: K. pneumoniae; S. pyogenes; M. tuberculosis.

Gram-negative bacteria: P. aeruginosa; E. coli; Proteus spp.

Details of organisms which may act as 'opportunist' causes of pneumonia in patients with immunodeficiencies are dealt with elsewhere.

FACTORS WHICH PREDISPOSE TO PNEUMONIA

1. *Viral Infections.* The respiratory viruses including influenza viruses, respiratory syncytial virus, rhinoviruses and adenoviruses as well as *varicella* (chickenpox), measles and smallpox viruses may all occasionally cause primary pneumonias but secondary bacterial invasion is the usual cause of pneumonias following the respiratory mucosal damage with these viruses.

2. *Chronic Airways Diseases.* Chronic bronchitis, bronchiectasis and cystic fibrosis all predispose to pneumonia usually caused by bacteria such as *H. influenzae, P. aeruginosa* and *Proteus.*

3. *Bronchial Obstruction.* Pneumonia secondary to bronchial obstruction by carcinoma, foreign bodies or benign tumours may occur and retention of secretions may lead to pneumonia following anaesthesia or drug and alcohol abuse.

4. *Aspiration Pneumonia.* This may occur in the unconscious patient and also to oesophageal disorders including hiatus hernia, achlasia of the cardia, systemic sclerosis (scleroderma), oesophageal diverticula and carcinomas.

5. *Impaired Resistance.* In addition to immunodeficiencies which are dealt with elsewhere, pneumonia is said to occur more commonly in patients suffering from malnutrition, uncontrolled diabetes mellitus, rheumatoid arthritis and chronic renal disease.

Clinical Features of Pneumonia. The physical signs and systemic upset may vary considerably. Some or all of the characteristic features may be modified by treatment or may be absent especially in the very young and old.

1. NON-SPECIFIC FEATURES. These include malaise, fever (38–40°C) rigors, vomiting, confusion and disorientation due to hypoxia which is especially common in the elderly. In severe cases dehydration, hypotension and delirium may follow.

2. RESPIRATORY FEATURES. Breathlessness, tachypnoea, pleuritic chest pain and cough which may be unproductive at first and later followed by haemoptysis. In classic pneumococcal pneumonia the sputum has a characteristic rusty tinge due to the presence of altered blood. The patient may appear cyanosed with short grunting respirations if there is pleurisy. Signs of consolidation may be late in appearance and in bronchopneumonia the only abnormal signs in the chest may be crackles on auscultation.

3. CARDIOVASCULAR FEATURES. There is usually a tachycardia and atrial fibrillation or flutter are common. Signs of heart failure may develop especially at the extremes of age. Hypotension may occur with dehydration or as an effect of the infection especially with Gram-negative organisms.

SPECIAL FEATURES

1. *Streptococcus pneumoniae.* Lobar pneumonia is now uncommon but *S. pneumoniae* is still the commonest organism to cause pneumonia. Infection is common in the young and elderly and as a complication of chronic bronchitis. Most strains of the organism are penicillin sensitive but an increasing incidence of resistance to tetracyclines has been observed. Septicaemia is particularly likely to occur with the Type III pneumococcus.

2. *Mycoplasma pneumoniae.* This is especially likely to affect older children and young adults amongst whom it is now the commonest cause of pneumonia. Infections with this organism commonly occur in epidemics, the majority of affected individuals have minor respiratory illnesses and cases of pneumonia are scattered sporadically through the affected population. Headache and mild fever (38–39°C) often precede the respiratory symptoms. Cough which is distressing but unproductive is a prominent and often persistent symptom. The physical signs in the chest may be limited to a few localized crackles but the chest X-ray appearances are usually more extensive and are often unilateral in distribution. A number of associated features are found in a minority of patients. These include erythema multiforme and other skin rashes, myringitis, polyarthropathy, meningo-encephalitis and aseptic meningitis. Although about half the patients who have mycoplasma pneumonia develop cold agglutinins in their serum, less than 5 per cent develop an associated haemolytic anaemia.

3. *Staphylococcal pneumonia.* This may occur in previously healthy people at times of influenza epidemics. It is common in drug addicts using intravenous drugs and may occur in patients with chronic lung diseases. Lung abscess and empyema are common sequelae and many of these organisms are resistant to penicillin.

4. *Klebsiella pneumoniae.* This is a rare but dangerous cause of

pneumonia with a high mortality. The patient is usually severely ill and sputum is scanty but bloodstained. Bronchiectasis, lung abscess and empyema are common sequelae.

5. *Rickettsia burnetti.* This organism is usually found in cattle and sheep but in man may cause an atypical pneumonia with marked headache and muscle pains. The duration of the illness is relatively short but the incubation period is long (28 days) so that a contact history may be overlooked.

6. *Chlamydia psittaci.* The psittacosis-ornithosis group of viruses may cause a severe pneumonia with a high mortality. The infection is acquired by contact with birds, especially parrots and pigeons.

Investigations and Diagnosis. Circumstantial features alone may be misleading so an attempt at a microbiological diagnosis must always be made.

MICROBIOLOGY. This should be attempted but may be unsuccessful. Sometimes blood cultures may yield the causative organism. Immediate Gram and Ziehl—Neelsen stains of sputum can be very helpful, thus: *S. pneumoniae* may be identified as Gram-positive diplococci; staphylococci appear as clusters of Gram-positive cocci; and if acid-fast bacilli are present they are most likely to be *M. tuberculosis.* Gram-negative organisms may be contaminants or genuine pathogens and other evidence will be necessary to make the distinction. If it is difficult to obtain *sputum* try simple physiotherapy and postural drainage. Invasive techniques are justified for seriously ill patients, those with immunological deficiencies, or those who fail to respond to treatment. Available techniques include *tracheal aspiration* through the cricothyroid membrane; *fibreoptic bronchoscopy* using a fine flexible cannula for suction or *transbronchial lung biopsy* with fluoroscopic control. *Percutaneous needle puncture* of lung with a lumbar puncture needle may be useful in severely ill patients. In addition to routine bacteriological culture, specimens should be sent for anaerobic culture and special methods for identification of fungi and *Pneumocystis carinii* in immunodeficient patients.

PLEURA. An overt pleural effusion should always be aspirated and the fluid stained and cultured for micro-organisms.

BLOOD INVESTIGATIONS. Total and differential white blood counts are useful. A total WBC below $10 \cdot 0 \times 10^9 / l$ suggests a viral or *M. pneumoniae* infection but in the first few days of bacterial infection and especially in the elderly or debilitated the total count may be low. A relative lymphocytosis may occur in viral infections or tuberculosis. A polymorph neutrophil leucocytosis is likely in bacterial infection and counts above $20 \cdot 0 \times 10^9 / l$, if sustained, suggest that an empyema or lung abscess may have developed.

SEROLOGICAL TESTS. An early blood sample is essential for comparison for later recognition of rising antibody titres to infection with influenza viruses *M. pneumoniae, C. psittaci* and *C. burnetti*. A fourfold or greater rise in titre after 14—21 days is taken as diagnostic of infection. Cold agglutinins appear in the first week after *M. pneumoniae* infection in 50 per cent of patients but haemolytic anaemia occurs only in about 1 in 10 of these. A raised ESR is common to most types of pneumonia, values above 50 mm/hr are common in *M. pneumoniae* infections. Additional investigations of value in more seriously ill patients include measurements of blood urea and electrolytes, blood gas tensions and liver function tests.

RADIOLOGICAL FEATURES. The causative agent may occasionally be correctly inferred from the chest X-ray appearances and history of the patient. *Lobar shadowing* with no displacement of the fissures is common in pneumococcal pneumonia. A *lobar or segmental shadow* with collapse suggests bronchial obstruction from carcinoma, foreign body or mucus impaction, and infection with mixed organisms is likely. *Multiple apical shadows* with cavitation, calcification and fibrotic shadows suggests tuberculosis. *Hazy 'ground-glass' shadowing* with few physical signs in the chest occurs in *M. pneumoniae* or viral infections. *Cavitation within patchy shadows* is likely to be staphylococcal pneumonia or due to Gram-negative or anaerobic organisms. *Bilateral patchy shadowing* with pre-existing lung disease in young or elderly patients may be due to infection with *S. pneumoniae*, or staphylococci. With *unilateral basal shadowing* and a pleural effusion, always consider a subphrenic cause and mixed infection including Gram-negative organisms. *Patchy shadowing* with cystic areas occurs with bronchiectasis and mixed infections including staphylococci and *P. aeruginosa* are usual.

ELECTROCARDIOGRAM. This may be necessary for the identification of any dysrhythmias which may develop but a prospective recording at the outset is advisable in assessing those patients who may have underlying heart disease.

Management. Uncomplicated pneumonia in an otherwise healthy patient can be treated at home. Admission to hospital is advisable when the patient is very ill or for secondary pneumonias in patients with asthma, chronic bronchitis, bronchiectasis, or cystic fibrosis and for those with generalized systemic diseases or those whose home circumstances are unsatisfactory.

GENERAL MEASURES. Bed rest is only necessary for the very ill. A general diet is suitable for those with any appetite and in most cases fluid balance can be maintained by oral fluids, otherwise intravenous saline and dextrose should be used. Hypoxia should be treated with oxygen. If the arterial carbon dioxide tension is normal or low a high oxygen concentration (<60 per cent) may be given by mask. For those patients with respiratory failure and carbon dioxide retention low concentrations of oxygen (24 or 28 per cent) should be given through a Venturi mask. Fluid retention due to heart failure should be treated with diuretics, starting with frusemide 40 mg by intravenous injection if a rapid response is needed. Continuation therapy with a suitable thiazide diuretic is usually adequate. Potassium supplements should always be given.

RELIEF OF PAIN AND COUGH. Painful cough may often be relieved by inhalation of moist aerosols or more simply with Friar's Balsam inhalations. Pleuritic pain may be relieved with dihydrocodeine tartrate (DF118). Linctus codeine (BNF) or pholcodeine (BPC) may serve a dual purpose of relieving pain and cough. Where these are ineffective pentazocine hydrochloride should be tried. Only in extreme cases should pethidine or morphine be used because of the potential hazard of respiratory depression.

ANTIBIOTIC THERAPY. This should be started as soon as specimens have been obtained for culture. *Table* 4 shows the range of activity of the available antibiotics.

PRIMARY PNEUMONIA. Although *S. pneumoniae* is still the most likely cause of lobar pneumonia and benzylpenicillin would be highly potent against that organism most physicians would now prefer to use a more broad-spectrum antibiotic especially if the pneumonia is severe in previously healthy patients. Amoxycillin 0·5 g 6-hourly, ampicillin 1·0 g 6-hourly or co-trimoxazole two tablets three times daily would all be suitable. Previously tetracycline would have been equally suitable but increasing numbers of strains of *S. pneumoniae* are reported resistant to the tetracyclines.

In patients with chronic bronchitis and asthma, lobar, segmental or more widespread pneumonia is usually caused by *S. pneumoniae* or *H. influenzae* and amoxycillin or ampicillin in the above doses are suitable treatment. True primary viral pneumonia is uncommon but secondary bacterial invasion with these same organisms commonly follows initial lung injury by influenza and other virus infections. Where the patient is sensitive to penicillin, erythromycin, clindamycin or co-trimoxazole are suitable substitutes. Gram stains of sputum may be invaluable in guiding the choice of antibiotic in this group of patients. If clumps of Gram-positive cocci are found the presence of penicillin-resistant staphylococci is a strong possibility and flucloxacillin should be added to the other antibiotics. For patients with penicillin hypersensitivity sodium fusidate (Fucidin), minocyclin (Minocin) or lincomycin (Lincocin) are suitable substitutes. Staphylococcal pneumonia may occur in previously healthy

Table 4. Choice of antibiotic therapy

Organism	First Choice	Other Suitable Drugs
S. pneumoniae *S. pyogenes*	Benzylpenicillin	Erythromycin, oxytetracycline, Cephalosporins
S. pyogenes i. Penicillin sensitive	Benzylpenicillin	
ii. Penicillin resistant	Cloxacillin, flucloxacin or methicillin plus benzylpenicillin	Cephalosporin Fusidic acid, erythromycin, lincomycin, clindamycin
H. influenzae	Ampicillin, amoxycillin	Oxytetracycline, co-trimoxazole, chloramphenicol
K. pneumoniae	Streptomycin plus oxytetracycline	Cephalosporins, chloramphenicol
E. coli	Check sputum sensitivities	Oxytetracycline, cephalosporins, carbenicillin, kanamycin
P. mirabilis	Check sputum sensitivities	Ampicillin, cephalosporins, carbenicillin, chloramphenicol, kanamycin
P. aeruginosa	Check sputum sensitivities	Gentamicin plus carbenicillin, tobramycin, colistin
M. pneumoniae	Oxytetracycline	Erythromycin
R. burnetti *Chlamydia*	Oxytetracycline Oxytetracycline	
Bacteroids etc.	Check sputum sensitivities. Penicillin, metronidazole co-trimoxazole	
Legionnaires' bacterium (?)	Erythromycin	

people during influenza epidemics and more often in patients with bronchiectasis or cystic fibrosis and drug addicts.

Mycoplasma pneumoniae, Chlamydia psittaci and *Rickettsia burnetti* are sensitive to tetracyclines and erythromycin but treatment is probably still best begun with ampicillin or amoxycillin unless there is strong circumstantial evidence to suspect a non-bacterial infection. If there is no response to treatment in 5–7 days, change to tetracycline 0·5 g 6-hourly. In children and pregnant women where tetracyclines are contraindicated because they stain teeth and bones and in patients hypersensitive to tetracyclines, erythromycin or co-trimoxazole is the drug of choice for *M. pneumoniae* infection.

ASPIRATION PNEUMONIA. Following coma or resulting from oeso-phageal abnormalities, is usually caused by mixed infection with anaerobic organisms including Gram-positive cocci, fusobacteria and bacteroides in addition to aerobic organisms. Benzylpenicillin is the drug of first choice for anaerobic organisms but for penicillin-resistant strains of bacteroides other antibiotics which are useful are clindamycin, chloramphenicol and metronidazole. In hospital aspiration pneumonias are most likely to be caused by Gram-negative organisms or *S. aureus,* and the addition of gentamicin and fluc-loxacillin, respectively, to benzylpenicillin is advisable. Infection with *P. aeruginosa* is. likely to occur in patients in hospital, especially those treated with respirators or humidifiers. The most effective combination is carbenicillin by intravenous injection and gentamicin by intramuscular injection. Tobramycin by intravenous infusion is suitable for Gram-negative infections of this type. *Secondary bacterial pneumonias in patients with systemic disease* including renal failure, heart failure, rheumatoid arthritis and collagen diseases is commoner than in normal people and whether infection has begun at home or in hospital the criteria for choosing antibiotics are similar to those for other patients. *Patients with congenital or acquired immunoglobulin deficiencies* are prone to bacterial infections. Pneumococcal pneumonia is common and Gram-negative pneumonias are frequently seen in patients with multiple myelomatosis. Oropharyngeal sepsis with spread to the lungs is common in patients with deficient or defective polymorphonuclear leucocytes. Immunodeficiency caused by disease or by corticosteroid or other treatment is associated with increased susceptibility to bacterial and other opportunist organisms including fungi, viruses and protozoa (*see* Chapter 15).

VERY SEVERE PNEUMONIA. Where patients with pneumonia are severely ill with hypotension, cyanosis and marked systemic upset it is advisable to try to get sputum and blood cultures first and then to treat promptly with antibiotics effective against pneumococci, streptococci, penicillinase-resistant staphylococci and *K. pneumoniae* until the causative organisms have been isolated. A suitable antibiotic combination would be benzylpenicillin 2 mega-units 6-hourly, flucloxacillin 1 g i.v. and then 0·5 g 6-hourly and gentamicin 1 mg per kg body weight 8-hourly or tobramycin 120 mg 8-hourly. For penicillin-sensitive patients cephaloridine 1 g 8-hourly or lincomycin 600 mg 8-hourly by i.v. infusion should be substituted for flucloxacillin. In addition to these measures i.v. fluid replacement and corticosteroids may be necessary in the hypotensive, severely shocked patient.

Antibiotic therapy should always be continued for a minimum of 5 days and until the patient has been afebrile for 48 hours. For the severely ill patient treatment for 7–10 days is advisable and for destructive pneumonias with staphylococcal or klebsiella infection several weeks' treatment may be advisable. Antibiotic therapy should not be changed for at least 48 hours and only if there is no clinical improvement.

LEGIONNAIRES' DISEASE. This form of severe pneumonia was first recognized and named from an outbreak with many deaths which occurred among delegates at an American Legion congress. Cases have since been reported from European countries, including Britain. The clinical features include a prodromal illness with malaise, muscle aches, mounting fever and rigors. This is followed by profound respiratory failure often requiring mechanical ventilation. Death has occurred in about 20 per cent of cases from cardiovascular collapse and sometimes renal failure. Sputum is usually scanty and not frankly purulent and pathogens have not been isolated from blood or sputum. The white blood count is usually normal or slightly raised. The chest X-ray shows patchy shadowing which is unilateral in about half the cases. At postmortem the lungs show changes of a bacterial pneumonia with alveolar damage. In a few cases a Gram-negative bacillus has been recovered from the lungs at post-mortem. Lung tissue injected into guinea-pigs causes death within a few days and large numbers of the bacillus can then be recovered from the animals. At present the simplest and most reliable test confirming the diagnosis is the demonstration of a fourfold or greater rise in titre of serum immunofluorescent antibody to the Legionnaires' bacillus or a positive titre of greater than 1/120–1/256. Legionnaires' disease should be suspected in any patient with severe pneumonia which fails to respond to conventional antibiotic therapy. Erythromycin is the most effective drug against Legionnaires' bacillus but tetracyclines have been successful in some cases.

Chapter 13

PULMONARY TUBERCULOSIS

Primary Tuberculosis; Postprimary Tuberculosis; Pleural Tuberculosis; Miliary Tuberculosis; Tuberculosis complicating other diseases.

Tuberculosis is still a major cause of morbidity and mortality especially in underdeveloped countries. There are about 10 million cases of active tuberculosis and 3 million deaths each year throughout the world. In some Asian countries 1 per cent or more of the population may have positive sputum smears for *Mycobacterium tuberculosis*. In the UK as in other developed countries there has been a steady fall in mortality and morbidity from tuberculosis, firstly as a result of improved nutrition, living conditions and public health measures, and more recently due to effective chemotherapy. There are still about 10 000 new notifications of tuberculosis each year in the UK and although there was a decline in notification rates of 43 per cent between 1965 and 1971 in indigenous subjects, there has been a rise of 68 per cent among Asian-born immigrants and the rate is more than 70 times higher in Pakistani immigrants compared with British-born subjects. Asian immigrants now contribute about 25 per cent of all new notifications. About 1500 deaths from tuberculosis are still recorded each year in England and Wales and some 20 per cent of these are not recognized until post-mortem. This is particularly a problem in elderly patients and although the notifications have fallen in other age groups, there has been little change in the notification rate in elderly males since the introduction of chemotherapy.

Control Measures. Pasteurization of milk and tuberculin testing of cattle had largely eradicated bovine infection in the UK but recently badgers in the West Country have been identified as a reservoir of infection. Mass miniature radiography has now been withdrawn because of the low prevalence of tuberculosis but is still useful in special high-risk groups in mental hospitals, prisons, vagrants' lodging houses, immigrants and contacts of infectious patients. Mass tuberculin testing is still carried out in British schoolchildren at 11 years of age and is useful as a means to select those where BCG vaccination may be helpful. BCG will confer 80 per cent protection against tuberculosis for about fifteen years, but with the declining attack rate the use of BCG in low-risk groups is not now likely to be valuable. In the UK primary chemoprophylaxis, i.e. treatment of uninfected tuberculin-negative individuals to prevent tuberculous infection, is generally reserved for infants of sputum-positive mothers. Secondary chemoprophylaxis, i.e. treatment of infected tuberculin-positive individuals to prevent clinical disease, is advisable for children under 5 with strongly positive tuberculin reactions and older children recently in contact with infectious tuberculosis to prevent them developing tuberculous meningitis and for anyone showing tuberculin conversion at any age. Patients with calcified pulmonary shadows on long-term corticosteroid therapy are probably best observed and not given chemoprophylaxis.

Pathology. The primary tuberculous lesion is subpleural and the upper zones are most commonly affected. Tubercle bacilli deposited in an alveolus are surrounded by a serous or serofibrinous exudate with neutrophils which are later replaced by macrophages to form a tubercle. This is a granulomatous lesion containing epithelioid cells (macrophages), Langhans giant cells with multiple nuclei (derived from macrophages), lymphocytes and a variable degree of fibrosis. Central necrosis produces macroscopic caseation and if the material is later discharged into the airways, cavitation will result. The primary lesion may heal by fibrosis but viable dormant tubercle bacilli may remain for years. If active progression occurs, infection may spread by local extension, lymph channels and through the blood.

Evolution of Tuberculous Infection. The development of classic tuberculous infection is rarely seen in the UK since the introduction of effective chemotherapy. Infection results from inhalation of tubercle bacilli from an infected individual and usually occurs following close contact and heavy exposure. The primary pulmonary infection with *M. tuberculosis* develops within four weeks and lymph glands at the hilum are usually involved. This may be symptomless, or occasionally give rise to a non-specific febrile illness and sometimes erythema nodosum. The tuberculin test becomes positive and if healing occurs, a degree of immunity to the tubercle bacillus develops. The peripheral lung lesion becomes calcified and may remain visible on chest X-ray as a Ghon focus. *If the disease progresses* extension in the same lobe of the lung leads to cavitation. Spread to the rest of the lung can lead to bilateral tuberculous bronchopneumonia. Pleural involvement with microscopic lesions causing a pleural effusion may develop within 3–6 months of infection in adolescents or young adults but is rare in children under 5.

Progression by lymphatic infection with lymph-node enlargement may compress the trachea or bronchi. Subsequent erosion and inhalation of infected material will lead to further spread. Lobar distension due to partial obstruction of a bronchus can cause localized emphysema. If spread occurs via the blood stream infection may develop in bone, kidney, adrenals, brain and meninges, and rarely miliary tuberculosis may develop.

Postprimary Tuberculosis. This may result from a progression of the primary lesion, but usually in the UK it occurs due to re-activation of the primary lesion, commonly in middle-aged and elderly men. This may be the result of impaired immunity from poor nutrition, secondary to other disease or as a result of treatment with immunosuppressants. The speed of progress, extent of infection and healing by fibrosis vary widely and a broad range of appearances from rapid caseating pneumonia and extensive bronchopneumonia to irregular areas of cavitation and chronic circumscribed fibrotic infection may be seen.

Clinical Features. Uncomplicated primary pulmonary tuberculosis is often symptomless in older children or adults, but in younger children constitutional symptoms are usual. Erythema nodosum may develop within a few weeks of tuberculous infection. Compression of the trachea or main bronchi from lymph-node enlargement may cause breathlessness, stridor and paroxysmal cough and partial bronchial obstruction acting as a check-valve may cause localized emphysema through overinflation.

Many patients may be symptom-free. Common presentations are: the middle-aged patient with persistent cough and purulent sputum; unexplained haemoptysis; unresolved pneumonia; non-specific symptoms including fever; malaise and weight loss. These are particularly likely to occur in Asian immigrants and tuberculosis is especially likely to escape notice in the elderly.

Physical Signs. The possible combinations of physical signs in patients with tuberculosis are legion. It is common for there to be few abnormal signs on examination, even in the presence of advanced disease. Wheezing, stridor, signs of consolidation and persistent inspiratory and expiratory crackles, especially over the upper lobes are all frequently observed in patients with tuberculosis.

Radiological Features. There are many patterns of change to be seen on X-ray with active tuberculosis. Common amongst these are:
1. Patchy solid lesions of a part of one lobe or lung.
2. Cavitated solid lesions.
3. Areas of streaky fibrosis.
4. Irregular areas of calcification. These may be suggestive of previous tuberculous infection but it is not possible to discount active infection even with calcified shadows.
5. Solitary round shadows are a frequent diagnostic problem in respiratory medicine and differentiation between a tuberculoma and a neoplasm may only be possible after resection of the lesion.
6. Hilar lymph-gland enlargement, especially in association with a lung lesion, may be characteristic of tuberculosis but again depending upon the age of the patient differentiation from bronchial carcinoma or lymphoma may require extensive investigation.
7. Pleural effusion. This is now rare in the UK. It usually develops within 3–6 months of the initiation of primary infection.

Symptoms. Include pleuritic pain, malaise with persistent fever.

Persistent cough in a middle-aged smoker should never be attributed to cigarette smoking without chest X-ray and clinical examination to exclude causes other than simple bronchitis.

Gastrointestinal symptoms such as anorexia and dyspepsia. Patients with peptic ulcer, especially those who have had a total gastrectomy show an increased susceptibility to pulmonary tuberculosis. Long-term corticosteroid and other immunosuppressive therapy may lead to reactivation of old lesions and such patients should have regular chest X-rays. Miliary spread and spontaneous pneumothorax are rare presentations of tuberculosis.

MILIARY TUBERCULOSIS. Haematogenous spread of tuberculosis is especially likely to occur in very young children, in the elderly and in those suffering from other diseases especially where the immunological defences are impaired. The chest X-ray is often normal.

Diagnosis of Tuberculosis. Investigation is frequently undertaken because of X-ray appearances which are suggestive of tuberculosis.

BACTERIOLOGY. The diagnosis is based on the finding of tubercle bacilli in the sputum. At least three sputum smears, laryngeal swabs or gastric aspirates should be examined by direct smear with fluorescent microscopy or Ziehl—Neelson staining. Culture and examination is still necessary in the UK to recognize atypical mycobacteria which account for 1–2 per cent of infections at present, and the incidence of primary resistant organisms may increase due to the present frequency of infection in Asian immigrants. Cultures take 4–7 weeks and in vitro sensitivity testing to antituberculous drugs requires a further three weeks.

BIOPSY. When suitable biopsy material is available, the diagnosis of tuberculosis can be made rapidly. With fibreoptic bronchoscopy it is easy to obtain mucosal or lung tissue for histology and culture.

TUBERCULIN TESTING. Within 3–4 weeks from initial infection hypersensitivity to tubercle bacillus proteins develops and can be demonstrated by intradermal injection of purified protein derivative (PPD). This cell-mediated (Gell and Coombs Type IV) response forms a raised area of induration with associated erythema.

The World Health Organization standard is still the Mantoux test. If infection is suspected begin with one tuberculin unit (1 TU) as 0·1 ml of 1/10 000 PPD. The result is read at 48–72 hours and erythema is discounted. A positive reaction, evidence of present or past infection with *M. tuberculosis,* is an area of induration of at least 10 mm diameter to 5 TU. Lesser degrees of reaction are regarded as non-specific. The multipuncture Heaf test and Tine test each using 5 TU, are widely used and are more convenient, but are less reliable. The Heaf test is read at 3–5 days and the confluent disc of induration is equivalent to a positive reaction to the Mantoux test. With the Tine test, 2–4 papules each at least 2 mm diameter constitutes a positive reaction.

Treatment of Tuberculosis. It is not essential to segregate patients with infectious (smear-positive) tuberculosis, but in Britain most patients are

Table 5. Drug treatment of tuberculosis

Drug	Dosage	Toxicity and Side Effects
First-line Drugs		
Streptomycin	1 g daily < 40 years 0·75 g daily > 40 years 1 g twice weekly with high dose isoniazid	8th cranial nerve vestibular damage. Deafness is rare Special caution in the elderly and renal insufficiency Allergic rashes and fever
Isoniazid	300 mg daily 15 mg/kg twice weekly with streptomycin	Toxic peripheral neuritis, in slow acetylators, prevented by pyridoxine Acute hepatic necrosis Sleeplessness, impaired memory and increased liability to epilepsy are uncommon side effects. Hypersensitivity is rare
Rifampicin	450–600 mg daily	Transient increase in serum transaminases is universal. Severe hepatotoxicity is uncommon. GI upsets, purpura and thrombocytopenia may occur. Brown red discoloration of urine is usual
Second-line drugs		
Pyrazinamide	40 mg/kg daily	Hepatotoxicity may be severe. Hyperuricaemia occasionally

Drug	Dose	Side effects
Thiacetazone	150 mg daily	Nausea, vomiting, giddiness, agranulocytosis and jaundice may occur with higher doses
PAS	12 g daily	GI irritation with nausea and vomiting or diarrhoea probably occur in 20 per cent of patients. Hypersensitivity reactions; interference with thyroid metabolism may cause goitre and hypothyroidism
Ethambutol	25 mg/kg daily for 2 months 15 mg/kg daily	Main toxic effect is retrobulbar neuritis causing loss of visual acuity, tunnel vision and impaired colour vision. Rare with lower dose. Recovery usual if drug is immediately withdrawn. Hypersensitivity reactions are uncommon
Ethionamide Prothionamide	1 g daily	GI upsets common. Hepatotoxicity, mental disturbance and neuropathies may occur
Cycloserine	1 g daily	May cause epilepsy and mental disturbance
Capreomycin Viomycin Kanamycin	15 mg/kg daily or 4 – 5 mg/kg	Nephrotoxicity, hypokalaemia and ototoxicity are common

admitted to hospital for the start of chemotherapy although the risk of infecting contacts is minimal. Hospital treatment is essential for:

1. Very ill patients needing rest.
2. Drug-resistant tuberculosis, hypersensitivity reactions or drug toxicity.
3. Uncooperative patients with bad domestic or social circumstances, mental disturbance or alcoholism where close supervision is essential.

CHEMOTHERAPY (*Table* 5). Chemotherapy, initially with three drugs, followed by continuation therapy using two drugs should avoid bacterial resistance developing provided that two drugs are always given to which the organisms are susceptible. In the UK 93 per cent of patients with newly diagnosed tuberculosis have organisms fully sensitive to the standard drugs (streptomycin, isoniazid and PAS). Initial resistance to one of these drugs is found in 3 per cent and an initial resistance to rifampicin and ethambutol is rare except in immigrants.

CHEMOTHERAPY FOR NEWLY DIAGNOSED DISEASE. Initial triple therapy with rifampicin, isoniazid and streptomycin or rifampicin, isoniazid and ethambutol is continued until the sensitivities of pre-treatment cultures are available at about 8 weeks.

CONTINUATION THERAPY. With isoniazid and ethambutol or isoniazid and rifampicin is now most commonly used. Although very short course regimens are being developed current practice is to give a minimum of 9 months' treatment for non-cavitated disease and 12—18 months for cavitated disease and extrapulmonary tuberculosis. The main cause of failure of chemotherapy is irregular self-medication. It is advisable to carry out spot-checks on patients at hospital visits using urine samples. Rifampicin gives a red colour to the urine and isoniazid is detected by colorimetric tests. If there is any doubt about the reliability of the patient a supervised intermittent out-patient treatment should be adopted, e.g.

a. *Streptomycin with Isoniazid.* Twice-weekly streptomycin 1 g with isoniazid 15 mg/kg given to out-patients has the benefit of reducing drug toxicity and lowering the cost of treatment.

b. *Rifampicin and Isoniazid.* Again twice-weekly in combination has been used but adverse reactions to rifampicin including thrombocytopenia, purpura, liver damage and renal damage have been reported. At present such regimens are under evaluation and cannot be recommended for routine use.

CHEMOTHERAPY FOR RE-TREATMENT. Before planning treatment of patients with resistant organisms or a history of previous treatment failure it is essential to construct a detailed record of the patient's previous drug therapy and obtain fully reliable sensitivity tests on new cultures of the organisms. New drugs should never be added to a previously unsatisfactory regimen. Where rifampicin and ethambutol have not previously been given and the organisms are fully sensitive, these are the best drugs to use. Others are listed in *Table 5*. All are less effective and more toxic than the first-line drugs. In general as many as possible of the available drugs should be used, depending upon the results of initial sensitivity tests. Thereafter a combination of three, or, less satisfactorily, two drugs, should be continued for 18 months. Careful observation for toxicity is essential with reserve drugs.

SURGERY. It is only occasionally necessary to resect localized lesions, and open healed cavities after adequate chemotherapy do not require operation. Occasionally relief of bronchostenosis or the removal of localized areas of bronchiectasis may be necessary.

INFECTION WITH OPPORTUNISTIC MYCOBACTERIA. At present about 1·5 per cent of all primary cultures in the UK grow atypical mycobacteria. The commonest organism isolated is *Mycobacterium Kansasii*. More rarely *M. scrofulaceum* or *M. intracellulare* may be obtained, most commonly from tuberculous adenitis. Many of these opportunistic mycobacteria are resistant *in vitro* to antituberculous drugs, but fortunately *M. Kansasii* shows a better response to treatment than the others. Before starting chemotherapy it is advisable to be sure that these organisms are not merely present as contaminants rather than truly acting as pathogens. Careful clinical assessment is necessary. Patients affected are commonly middle-aged or elderly men and predisposing factors include dusty occupations, chronic bronchitis, emphysema and pneumoconiosis. Where localized disease is unresponsive to antituberculous drugs surgical resection should be considered.

ADVERSE DRUG REACTIONS

Allergic reactions are commonest with PAS and streptomycin and usually occur within the first six weeks of treatment. The commonest encountered are fever, rash and pruritus. Less common reactions include lymphadenopathy, hepatosplenomegaly, liver damage, proteinuria, encephalopathy, transient lung shadows, eosinophilia and blood dyscrasias. The offending drug is identified by stopping all treatment and then giving small test doses of each drug in turn. Thereafter management is as follows. Either:

    a. Replace the offending drug.

    b. Hyposensitization to the drug, giving at least two other effective drugs to prevent the emergence of drug resistance.

    c. Suppression of the allergic reaction by corticosteroids.

Toxic reactions are also common. The following are the commonest encountered in practice:

Streptomycin. In general toxicity is related to blood levels and renal function should always be checked before starting treatment. It is possible to use streptomycin in the presence of impaired renal function provided the blood levels are carefully monitored.

Isoniazid. Rarely causes toxicity in the conventional dose of 300 mg per day. With intermittent treatment in larger doses peripheral neuropathy may occur, especially in alcoholics and children. A small daily dose of pyridoxine 10 mg will protect against nerve damage. Very rarely hepatotoxicity occurs.

Rifampicin. May be hepatotoxic and liver function tests should always be checked *before* starting treatment. With normal hepatic function transient elevation of serum enzymes occurs during the first two or three weeks' treatment with rifampicin but severe liver damage is rare. Rifampicin enhances liver microsomal enzyme activity increasing the metabolism of a number of drugs including oral contraceptives, so that women taking rifampicin should use other forms of contraception.

Ethambutol. May cause retrobulbar neuritis but this is rare with the the lower dose of 15 mg/kg daily. Ophthalmalogical examination should precede treatment but thereafter regular visual acuity tests are unnecessary. The patient should be warned to discontinue the drugs at the first sign of any visual impairment.

Corticosteroids. These have no beneficial effect on the degree of pulmonary fibrosis or the speed of sputum conversion but are indicated for:

   a. Desperately ill patients to produce rapid reduction in fever.
   b. To suppress severe drug allergy.
   c. They may possibly enhance recovery from large tuberculous pleural effusions.

BACTERIOLOGICAL CONTROL OF THERAPY. In the UK pretreatment sensitivity tests are of very limited value and routine sensitivity tests during treatment are unnecessary. It is common to find resistant cultures before sputum conversion during successful chemotherapy. Sputum smears and culture should be made monthly until smears are negative and thereafter at 2–3 monthly intervals.

A consistent rise in the number of acid-fast bacilli seen on direct smear during treatment indicates that the patient has stopped taking the drug or drug resistance has been acquired. However, at the beginning of treatment with regimens containing rifampicin it is common for large quantities of dead bacilli to be shed in the sputum. Sensitivity tests should be reserved for investigation of bacteriological relapse and in re-treatment.

CHEST RADIOGRAPHY. This is of limited value as a guide to progress during treatment and greater weight should be placed on the results of sputum cultures.

Chapter 14

FUNGAL INFECTIONS OF THE LUNG

INCIDENCE

These uncommon infections have characteristic clinical presentations which must be recognized.

Pulmonary mycoses endemic to the UK include *Aspergillosis, Candidiasis, Actinomycosis, Nocardiosis* and *Cryptococcosis*. As a result of increased foreign travel occasional cases of *Histoplasmosis, Blastomycosis* and *Coccidioidomycosis* may also be seen.

Most infections seen in Britain are opportunist in that they occur in patients with defences impaired through malnutrition, lymphomas, leukaemia, multiple myeloma, sarcoidosis, tuberculosis or from treatment with antibiotics, corticosteroids or immunosuppressive agents.

ASPERGILLOSIS

This is the commonest of the pulmonary mycoses in Britain and is usually caused by infection with *Aspergillus fumigatus* but others of the species may occasionally infect man. It is a filamentous saprophytic fungus producing airborne spores and infection occurs through inhalation.

Types of Disease
1. ALLERGIC BRONCHOPULMONARY ASPERGILLOSIS. This is caused by Type I and Type III (Gell and Coombs) allergic reaction to the fungus.
2. INVASIVE ASPERGILLOSIS. This is an opportunist infection presenting as a necrotizing pneumonia, sometimes with an empyema. Disseminated infection also occurs.
3. ASPERGILLOMA. A mycelium of *A. fumigatus* may grow in cavities already present in the lung from previous tuberculosis, bronchiectasis, sarcoidosis, pneumoconiosis, diffuse pulmonary fibrosis or apical fibrosis in ankylosing spondylitis.

Clinical Features
1. *Subclinical infection* can occur and may only be recognized by the presence of precipitins to *A. fumigatus* in serum.
2. *Allergic bronchopulmonary aspergillosis*. Features include asthma, chronic cough with sputum, obstruction of proximal bronchi with mucus plugs containing hyphae of *A. fumigatus*. Bronchiectatic changes develop in the affected bronchi and distal fibrosis occurs.

   If unrecognized, allergic bronchopulmonary aspergillosis may recur for years presenting with episodes of transient pulmonary infiltration with blood eosinophilia, wheezing, low grade fever and systemic symptoms such as muscle aches.

3. *Simple aspergilloma*. This may be discovered by chance on chest X-rays as a round shadow within a cavity already present. Recurrent haemoptysis, sometimes massive, may be a problem.

4. *Secondary bacterial infection* of an aspergilloma. This usually presents with fever and purulent sputum which is often very foul due to the presence of anaerobic and Gram-negative organisms. This may be a prostrating illness.

5. Some aspergillomas may give rise to a Type III antigen–antibody reaction with marked fever and constitutional upset.

Diagnosis

1. CHEST X-RAYS. The characteristic appearance of an *aspergilloma* is a dense round opacity lying within a cavity with a crescent of air above it ('halo' sign). The X-ray features of *invasive aspergillosis* are non-specific with bilateral patchy coarse shadows in the lung fields.

2. IMMUNOLOGICAL TESTS
   Agar Gel Precipitin Tests. A positive result may be obtained before X-ray changes are visible. Over 90 per cent of patients with aspergillomas give a positive result with a strong reaction because of the presence of the large antigen load in the aspergilloma. Weaker reactions occur with subclinical infections. In allergic aspergillosis the reaction is usually slight but still present in about 70–75 per cent of patients.

3. SKIN TESTS. Immediate (Type I) and delayed (Type (III)) reactions are usually demonstrable with allergic aspergillosis but they are uncommon with aspergillomas unless there is coexistent allergic bronchopulmonary aspergillosis.

Treatment

1. ALLERGIC BRONCHOPULMONARY ASPERGILLOSIS. This responds well to treatment with corticosteroids which may have to be continued indefinitely.

2. INVASIVE ASPERGILLOSIS. This should be treated with a combination of oral amphotericin B and inhalation of brilliant green (anhydroxystilbamidine).

3. SIMPLE ASPERGILLOMA. Surgical resection is only indicated if severe recurrent haemoptysis is a problem or if the aspergilloma enlarges to become invasive. Secondary infection usually responds to antibiotics.

ACTINOMYCOSIS

Lung infection with *Actinomyces israeli*, a branching filamentous anerobic Gram-positive organism occasionally present in the mouth, usually follows inhalation after dental extractions or other surgical procedures.

Clinical Features. The onset is insidious with fever, cough and sputum containing the fungus. Suppuration and haemoptysis may occur and pleuritic pain and empyema occasionally develop. If chest wall involvement occurs skin sinuses may discharge pus containing the typical 'sulphur' granules of the mycelium of *A. israeli*.

Treatment. Benzylpenicillin 10–12 million units daily for up to 6 months. Rarely lung damage may need surgical excision once the infection has been controlled.

CANDIDIASIS

Lung infection with *Candida albicans* usually only occurs with severe underlying disease or immunosuppression.
> BRONCHIAL CANDIDIASIS. This causes scanty mucoid sputum and cough.
> PULMONARY CANDIDIASIS. This is a more severe illness with cough, fever, haemoptysis, breathlessness, chest pain and sometimes a pleural effusion.

Treatment. Amphotericin B by inhalation and i.v. infusions. 5-Fluorocytosine has also been used successfully.

NOCARDIOSIS

Infection with *Nocardia asteroides,* an aerobic organism, causes a chronic granulomatous disease affecting the lungs and other organs in a similar manner to actinomycosis. This soil saprophyte is thought to infect through skin damage or by inhalation.

Clinical Features. These include fever, cough, breathlessness and haemoptysis. The mortality rate is high.

Treatment. Long-term high doses of sulphadimidine.

CRYPTOCOCCOSIS (Torulosis)

Cryptococcus neoformans is a yeast widely present in soil and pigeon droppings. Infection usually occurs in individuals with underlying debilitating illnesses.

Clinical Features. The commonest presentation is a subacute meningoencephalitis. Respiratory infections may develop as a mild self-limiting influenza-like illness or as a typical pneumonia with fever, productive cough, occasional haemoptysis and pleuritic pains.
> CHEST X-RAYS. May show a solitary opacity, a lung abscess or diffuse pulmonary infiltration.

Diagnosis. This is made by demonstrating the organism in sputum.

Treatment. Daily amphotericin B by i.v. infusion for several weeks.

HISTOPLASMOSIS (Cave Fever)

This is caused by infection with *Histoplasma capsulatum,* a saprophyte present in soil and the droppings of birds, chickens and bats. It is endemic in parts of the USA, especially the Mississippi valley. Infection occurs by inhalation of the spores and occasionally as an opportunist infection.

Clinical Features. The majority of cases of infection are asymptomatic and are discovered subsequently by the presence of rounded opacities with hilar gland enlargement on chest X-ray. These later become calcified. *Progressive disease.* This occurs in about 1 per cent of infections.

Clinical Features. Include fever, malaise, weight loss, chest pain and sometimes mucocutaneous granulomatous lesions, hepatosplenomegaly, adrenal gland involvement, anaemia and leucopenia.

Diagnosis. Made by sputum examination for the organism, the Histoplasmin skin test and the demonstration of rising titres of complement-fixing antibodies in serum.

Treatment. For the progressive disease consists of amphotericin B by intravenous infusion for 10–14 days.

COCCIDIOIDOMYCOSIS (Valley Fever)

This soil organism, *Coccidioidomycosis immitis,* is endemic in the West and South-West of the USA. Infection occurs by inhalation of the arthrospores. *Primary Infection.* Commonly this is asymptomatic but about half the affected patients show a subacute respiratory infection resembling viral pneumonia with fever, cough, chest pain, headache, sore throat and occasionally bloodstained sputum. Erythema nodosum and erythema multiforme occasionally occur together with joint pains. *Progressive Infection.* This is rare. It presents with weight loss, malaise, fever and breathlessness and other lung signs. Granulomatous reactions may be present in the brain, meninges, bone and skin.

Chest X-rays. This will show cavitation, solid rounded shadows, hilar lymph-gland enlargement and diffuse miliary shadowing in the progressive form of the disease.

The *coccidioidin skin test* will be positive in the majority of cases and a rising titre of complement-fixing antibodies will be found in serum. The organism may be identified in sputum smears.

Treatment. The progressive disease should be treated with intravenous amphotericin B for long periods.

BLASTOMYCOSIS (North American Blastomycosis)

The soil organism, *Blastomycosis dermitididis,* is endemic in the South-East USA.

Clinical Features. Ulcerative granulomas of the mouth and nasopharynx may be followed by invasive respiratory infection and pleural disease, not unlike tuberculosis, together with bone involvement and sinus formation. Constitutional upset is common.

Treatment. Amphotericin B for prolonged periods.

ANTIFUNGAL DRUGS

Amphotericin B (Fungilin; Fungizone). Although the most effective agent in most cases, it is difficult to administer. A total dose of 1 g of the drug over a period of 4 weeks is the minimum acceptable treatment and it is better to give up to 5 g in total. Higher doses may cause irreversible renal damage. Throughout treatment regular examination of renal function and urine should be made. The drug is usually given as a slow intravenous infusion in 5 per cent dextrose solution starting with a dose of 0·25 mg per kg per day increasing until the daily dose is 1 mg per kg per day. Nephrotoxicity may be reduced by simultaneous infusion of mannitol.

Fluorocytosine (Alcobon). This may be effective against *Candida albicans* and *Cryptococcus neoformans* but it is less effective overall, especially against aspergillus. It may be given by mouth in a dose of 200 mg per kg per day divided into 4 equal doses. Treatment should be carried on for several weeks.

Clotrimazole (Canesten). This is active against many fungi and yeasts in topical preparations. It is well absorbed from the gut but does cause gastrointestinal upsets. It is especially useful in systemic infections with candida or aspergillus. The dose is 70 mg per kg per day in divided doses.

Chapter 15

OPPORTUNIST LUNG INFECTIONS

Strictly speaking all infections are opportunistic, but this title is generally reserved for infection with organisms of unusual type or low pathogenicity in individuals with impaired defences. Factors contributing to opportunist infection are of two groups:

1. Basic diseases
   Neoplastic
   Immunodeficiency
      Primary
      Secondary
2. Additive factors
   a. Altered barriers:
       i. Catheters — intravenous, genito-urinary
       ii. IPPV and humidifiers
       iii. Tissue damage — gastrointestinal damage
   b. Altered flora — antibiotics
   c. Leucopenia
       Cytotoxics
       Radiotherapy
       Immunosuppressives
   d. Abnormality or reduction of leucocyte function
       Migration
       Phagocytosis
       Killing
   e. Impaired immunity B- or T-cell
       Steroids   Cytotoxics
       Radiotherapy   Antilymphocyte globulin

A careful history should include all details of recent treatment including drugs, radiotherapy and the possibility of exposure to known infections, e.g. influenza, *Mycoplasma pneumoniae*, *Varicella*. Physical examination may be unhelpful and classic signs such as fever may be absent or impaired. Unusual conditions like perirectal abscess should always be looked for. Cultures should be obtained of all available sites including the nose, throat, skin, faeces and urine, wounds, sputum, blood, intravenous catheters, cerebrospinal fluid and bone marrow. Blood tests should include a differential WBC, quantitative immunoglobulin levels, serum electrolytes, urea and blood sugar.

Diagnosis
   HISTORY to include:

    a. Drugs.
    b. Exposure to known infections.
PHYSICAL. Classic signs may be absent, especially fever – not diagnostic.
N.B. Perirectal abscess common with chemotherapy.
CULTURES From: nose; throat; skin; stool; urine; sputum; wound; blood (CSF and bone marrow).
BLOOD COUNT. Quantitative immunoglobulin levels; urea; electrolytes; blood sugar.

Specific Diseases which may impair Host Defence and lead to Opportunist Infections

1. *Congenital Bruton-type agammaglobulinaemia,* a rare primary inherited deficiency of B-cell function. These patients have deficient humoral defences and are subject to recurrent bacterial infection, e.g. pneumonia caused by *S. pneumoniae, S. pyogenes, P. aeruginosa* or *H. influenzae.* Cell-mediated immunity is intact and these subjects are not usually prone to viral and fungal infections. In the neoplastic diseases, immunodeficiencies of either B- or T-cell or a mixture of the two may occur.

2. *Hodgkin's disease:* Here T-cell immunity is deficient so viral infections are common especially with *Herpes simplex* or fungal and certain protozoal infections. Later B-cell deficiency may develop leading to pneumonias caused by *S. aureus, P. aeruginosa* or *Escherichia coli.* About 50 per cent of patients with Hodgkin's disease may develop primary or secondary pulmonary tuberculosis. In Hodgkin's disease pulmonary infiltration on chest X-ray is rarely due to infiltration of the lung by lymphoma unless hilar glands are also present. With clinical deterioration in the absence of proven bacterial disease possible causes include fungal infections, candidiasis or aspergillosis. With symptoms of nervous system involvement including headache or personality change, accompanied by chest X-ray evidence of lung involvement with well-circumscribed shadows 2–8 cm in diameter, *Cryptococcus neoformans* infection is a possible cause.

3. *Lymphosarcoma.* Involvement of the lungs and pleura is usually secondary to disease elsewhere and hilar lymph gland enlargement is rare. On chest X-ray secondary pulmonary lymphosarcoma presents as solitary or multiple nodules 3–8 cm in diameter. Secondary deposits of lymphosarcoma are usually endobronchial and may cause atelectasis and obstructive pneumonitis. The commonest immunodeficiency is of T-cell function so fungal and bacterial infections are common.

4. *The leukaemias.* About half of affected patients have enlarged mediastinal lymph glands and about 25 per cent have parenchymal involvement of the lungs at post-mortem but only about half of

either group are apparent on chest X-ray in life. The commonest X-ray appearances are hilar lymph-gland enlargement and bilateral diffuse reticular shadowing. Patients with chronic lymphatic leukaemia show both B- and T-cell deficiency and are prone to bacterial, viral and fungal infections. Cough, sputum and haemoptysis are more commonly caused by superimposed infection than leukaemic infiltration.

5. *Multiple myeloma.* Extension of the primary disease into the lungs is rare unless there is local involvement of a rib. The dominant immunodeficiency is of B-cell type predisposing to bacterial infections and in 75–80 per cent of cases the causative organism is Gram-negative. Infection with fungi and protozoa is uncommon.

6. *Primary bronchogenic carcinoma.* Lung shadows on chest X-ray early in the course of the disease may result from bacterial infection or by direct extension of the disease. Later, immunodeficiency may develop directly from the disease but it is more often due to treatment with radiotherapy or chemotherapy resulting in T-cell depletion with a predisposition to fungal and viral infections.

Management. If fever develops sputum, urine and other specimens should be taken for smears and cultures and treatment should begin with antibiotics. Of *fungal infections,* candidiasis and aspergillosis are the commonest encountered.

In all neoplastic diseases pulmonary shadowing may result from chemotherapy drugs, especially busulphan. Diffuse pulmonary fibrosis developing over a period of 3 or 4 years may present with cough or fever. Cyclophosphamide also causes pulmonary fibrosis while methotrexate may cause early reactions with fever, cough and breathlessness with bilateral diffuse shadowing. This may remit on stopping the drug. Bleomycin is another cause of early diffuse pulmonary fibrosis. Patients on immunosuppressive treatment commonly develop opportunist lung infections. Combination treatment with cytotoxic agents and corticosteroids will make patients prone to both T-cell and B-cell deficiencies and infections with bacteria, viruses and fungi are all common, including *Pneumocystis carinii, Cytomegalovirus, Aspergillus fumigatus* and *Candida albicans.*

Pneumocystis carinii infections present with two clinical patterns, either an insidious onset with cough and breathlessness leading to progressive dyspnoea and cyanosis with minimal fever or an acute onset with fever, headache, cough and breathlessness. In both forms chest X-rays may show bilateral perihilar nodular or reticulonodular shadowing. *Cytomegalovirus* infection usually involves the outer third of the lungs on chest X-ray with nodular shadows of 1-2 mm in diameter. *Candidiasis* and pulmonary *aspergillosis* present with cough, scanty sputum, pleuritic chest pain, airways obstruction and fever. The chest X-ray usually shows patches of dense shadowing (consolidation) without cavitation. The chest X-ray appearances may give a useful pointer to the cause of opportunist lung infections, *see Table* 6.

Table 6. Some characteristic chest X-ray appearances

1. Homogenous non-segmental or segmental shadows	
a with expansion of lobe (bulging fissures)	*Klebsiella* — *Aerobacter* or other Gram-negative organisms
b with rapid cavitation	Anaerobic organisms
2. Multiple masses, with or without cavitation	*a* fungi *b* staphylococci *c* *P. aeruginosa* *d* septic emboli *e* anaerobic organisms
3. Diffuse parenchymal disease	
a predominant acinar pattern	*Pneumocystis carinii* or mixed pathogens
b predominant reticular pattern	*Cytomegalovirus* or mixed pathogens

Investigations for Suspected Opportunist Infections

1. BRUSH BIOPSY. Good results have been recorded with *P. carinii* but the results have been more variable with other infections.
2. NEEDLE BIOPSY. Some studies have reported successful isolation of causative organisms in up to 75 per cent of cases. The dangers of this technique include haemoptysis and pneumothorax. Aspiration needle biopsy has been successful in diagnosis of *P. carinii* infections.
3. FIBREOPTIC BRONCHOSCOPY. Good results have been obtained with *P. carinii* infections, but less satisfactory results have been obtained with other types of infection.
4. OPEN BIOPSY. This remains the investigation of choice, where appropriate, when others have proved unsuccessful but it carries a higher risk of complications.

Table 7. Invasive investigations

1. *Brush Biopsy:*	*P. carinii* Other infections
2. *Needle Biopsy:*	Organisms recovered in 70–80 per cent cutting needles: haemoptysis may occur aspiration needle: good for *P. carinii*
3. *Fibreoptic bronchoscope:*	Good for *P. carinii* Other infections: results variable.
4. *Open Biopsy:*	Greater risks of complications.

Summary: The Approach to Opportunist Infections

1. Take all possible precautions to avoid infection, including nursing in isolation.
2. For B-cell deficiency remember that increased susceptibility to bacterial infection is common and notably patients with multiple myeloma and leukaemias are subject to B-cell deficiency.
3. T-cell deficiencies result in an increased susceptibility to viral and fungal infections but defences to bacterial infections are usually intact.
4. There are no truly unique clinical or radiological patterns to distinguish one infection from another, or to differentiate between lung infection and infiltration with neoplastic disease.
5. Examine and culture specimens from every possible source and site of infection.
6. Treat blindly with antibiotics *only* for presumed bacterial infection in leukaemias.
7. Open lung biopsy is the investigation of choice when all others have failed.

Chapter 16

DIFFUSE PULMONARY FIBROSIS

Sarcoidosis; Extrinsic Alveolitis; Drug-induced Lung Fibrosis; Pneumoconioses; Cryptogenic Fibrosing Alveolitis; Tuberous Sclerosis; Eosinophilic Granuloma; Rheumatoid Lung; Systemic Lupus Erythematosus; Scleroderma; Dermatomyositis.

Extensive fibrosis of the lungs, especially affecting the alveolar walls, may result from a number of diseases of widely differing aetiology including:

1. *Pulmonary granulomas,* sarcoidosis, berylliosis, extrinsic allergic alveolitis.
2. *Pulmonary exudates* may result from the following: raised left atrial pressure in mitral valve disease and hypertensive heart disease; chronic renal failure; chemical injury from vanadium, nitrous oxide, cadmium fumes, ozone; reaction to cytotoxic agents including busulfan and bleomycin; drug reactions to nitrofurantoin, salazopyrine, PAS; recurrent inhalation of gastric or oesophageal contents as with hiatus hernia and oesophageal strictures; inflammatory exudates to organisms; with adult respiratory distress syndrome, mechanism unknown but possibly immunological in type; with idiopathic haemosiderosis; systemic lupus erythematosus.
3. *Pneumoconioses,* silicosis, coal workers' pneumoconiosis, asbestosis.
4. *Diseases of unknown aetiology* including Hamman–Rich syndrome, cryptogenic fibrosing alveolitis, eosinophilic granuloma and tuberous sclerosis.

Pathology. As yet there are no known specific histological features of the various forms of diffuse pulmonary fibrosis which allow different diseases to be distinguished from each other. The granulomatous diseases tend to cause fibrosis predominantly in the connective tissues surrounding the airways, while pneumoconioses and fibrosing alveolitis show more marked effects in the alveolar walls. Many of the diseases are associated with 'desquamative' changes, i.e. the shedding of numbers of cells into the alveolar lumen including macrophages, mononuclear cells and altered Type II pneumonocytes with some intra-alveolar fibrosis. The other common histological feature, alveolar wall and inter-alveolar fibrosis with collagenous tissue is usually referred to as 'mural' change. There may be wide variation in the proportions of these two histological features found in different parts of the same lung.

Symptoms. Breathlessness is the commonest presenting complaint, first on effort, later at rest. Cough is common, usually unproductive and often distressing. In the later stages of all these diseases weight loss and fatigue are common.

121

Clinical Signs. *Finger Clubbing* is common in some diseases, e.g. asbestosis, cryptogenic fibrosing alveolitis, and rare in others, e.g. sarcoidosis. *Fine inspiratory crackles* at the lung bases due to closure of small airways are said to be more common in those diseases where the alveolar wall is predominantly affected, e.g. asbestosis, cryptogenic fibrosing alveolitis and less common in the granulomatous diseases, e.g. sarcoidosis, extrinsic alveolitis. Arterial desaturation with *cyanosis* is at first only present with exercise but later occurs at rest. In advanced disease right ventricular hypertrophy and right heart failure develop.

Physiological Effects. All lung volumes are reduced and in the absence of associated airways disease total lung volume and spirometric volumes (FEV_1 and FVC) are reduced in parallel without airways obstruction. The lungs are stiffer and so less compliant. Gas transfer is impaired mostly as a result of uneven distribution of ventilation and perfusion caused by the patchy nature of the disease. Initially hypoxia occurs without hypercapnia but when fibrosis becomes widespread carbon dioxide retention may also develop.

Radiological Changes. Although certain diseases tend to give characteristic patterns of pulmonary shadows any of these diseases can cause widespread irregular changes in lung markings. A few basic guidelines may be given:

> *Upper zones mainly affected*: silicosis, coal workers' pneumoconiosis, extrinsic allergic alveolitis.
>
> *Mid zones mainly affected:* sarcoidosis.
>
> *Lower zones mainly affected:* asbestosis and cryptogenic fibrosing alveolitis.
>
> *'Disappearing lung':* i.e. serial chest X-rays show progressive loss of size of the lung fields in scleroderma and systemic lupus erythematosus.
>
> *Honeycomb lung:* may occur with any of these diseases but is especially common with eosinophilic granuloma, tuberous sclerosis and rheumatoid lung.
>
> *Associated pleural plaques* occur with asbestosis.

Diagnosis and Investigations. The history is particularly important including a careful occupational history and details of previous drug treatment. Assessment of the duration and rate of progress of breathlessness, e.g. insidious onset and slow progress is common in pneumoconioses, more rapid progress tends to occur with cryptogenic fibrosing alveolitis. Other symptoms such as haemoptysis and sputum production suggest left ventricular failure or bronchiectasis. Involvement of other systems, e.g. arthritis, skin rashes occur with SLE and dermatomyositis. Although over 80 causes of diffuse pulmonary shadows have been described the list of possible causes in any patient can usually be narrowed to two or three.

CLINICAL PATTERNS

Subacute Illness with Fever, Breathlessness and Patchy Radiological Shadows. Causes include:

1. Organic dust diseases, including farmer's lung and bird fancier's lung.
2. Exposure to noxious gases such as ozone, nitrous oxide, cadmium fumes and halogens.
3. Inhalation of gastric or oesophageal contents.
4. Pneumonias, bacterial, viral or fungal.
5. Pulmonary eosinophilia, idiopathic, associated with allergic broncho-pulmonary aspergillosis or with drug reactions to sulphonamides, PAS, gold etc. Rarer causes include idiopathic pulmonary haemo-siderosis and Goodpasture's syndrome.

Another cause of breathlessness with patchy shadowing on chest X-ray which must be considered in this group is pulmonary oedema secondary to left ventricular failure.

Chronic Pulmonary Shadows without Fever. Causes to be considered include pneumoconioses, organic dust diseases, sarcoidosis, lipoid inhalation, carcinomatosis, extrinsic allergic alveolitis, cryptogenic fibrosing alveolitis.

Pulmonary Shadows with Multi-system Diseases. Diseases to be considered include ankylosing spondylitis, rheumatoid arthritis, systemic lupus erythematosus, scleroderma and dermatomyositis.

INVESTIGATIONS

1. *Sputum:* Smear and culture for tubercle bacilli, microscopy for eosinophils and asbestos bodies, cytological examination for malignant cells.
2. *Blood tests:* Full blood count and differential white cell count including eosinophils, rheumatoid factor, antinuclear factor, LE cells, ESR.
3. *Lung function tests and blood gases:* With and without exercise.
4. *Lung biopsy:* May sometimes be necessary, this will be discussed later.

SARCOIDOSIS

A systemic disease of unknown aetiology of world wide distribution commoner in northern Europe and amongst American Negroes, West Indians, and Irish immigrants. The prevalence in the UK is about 2 per 10 000 population. It commonly presents in the third and fourth decades but can occur at any age. The aetiology is unknown, probably it is a granulomatous response to a number of different factors amongst which may be mycobacteria. Affected individuals show defects of cellular immunity with depression of delayed hypersensitivity, e.g. to candida and PPD. Humoral immunity is not depressed and serum immunoglobulin levels may be high.

Pathology. The sarcoid granuloma consists of a group of large macrophages (epithelioid cells) and multinucleate giant cells surrounded by a scanty rim of lymphocytes. The giant cells have about 30 nuclei arranged peripherally with several types of inclusion bodies. Necrosis and calcification are rare and healing occurs with collagenous scar tissue. The disease usually affects several organs but the effects on one or two systems usually dominate the clinical picture. The sites most often involved are skin, lungs, lymph nodes, liver, spleen, bones, eyes and parotid glands. Lymph-node involvement is most commonly restricted to one or two groups. Rarely the central and peripheral nervous systems are affected.

Clinical Presentations. Pulmonary sarcoidosis usually presents as:

1. Chance detection of bilateral hilar lymphadenopathy on a routine chest X-ray with or without lung infiltration.
2. During investigation of non-respiratory symptoms of fever, eye involvement, skin lesions especially erythema nodosum.
3. Subacute respiratory illness with cough, chest pain, exertional dyspnoea, malaise or fever.

BILATERAL HILAR LYMPHADENOPATHY AND ERYTHEMA NODOSUM. Sarcoidosis is the commonest cause of erythema nodosum in young adults, often associated with acute arthritis of ankles, knees and wrists, acute anterior uveitis and parotid enlargement ('uveoparotid fever'). Low grade fever, lassitude, skin eruptions and joint pains are common. Differential diagnoses include tuberculosis and Hodgkin's disease. Clinical signs in the chest are usually scanty or absent.

DIFFUSE PULMONARY SHADOWS. These are usually present in association with bilateral hilar lymphadenopathy but may occur alone. Extensive pulmonary fibrosis develops in a minority of patients. Any fibrosis which has developed is probably not reversible, but treatment with corticosteroids can suppress further granuloma formation.

EXTRAPULMONARY MANIFESTATIONS

1. *Ocular Sarcoidosis.* Eye involvement occurs in about a quarter of all patients found to have sarcoidosis. Anterior uveitis is commonest with pain, misting of vision and reddening. Posterior uveitis is less common. Keratoconjunctivitis sicca and lacrimal gland involvement may occur with chronic disease.
2. *Skin Involvement.* Three main types of lesion occur:
   a. Discrete nodules, yellowish in colour with a dry scaly surface.
   b. Lupus pernio, large lobulated purple nodules usually on the hands or feet.

    c. Flat patches with granular or scaly surfaces on the trunk and extremities.

3. *Liver and Spleen.* Commonly involved in sarcoidosis. Hepatic involvement may be present in 70–85 per cent of patients with bilateral hilar lymphadenopathy.

4. *Bone Involvement.* Cystic lesions of bone affecting the hands and feet are uncommon.

5. *Nervous System.* Sarcoidosis affecting the nervous system is rare. The presentations most often seen include mononeuritis multiplex, focal cranial nerve lesions and meningeal involvement. Obscure neurological syndromes with epilepsy may also occur.

6. *Calcium Metabolism.* Hypercalcaemia and hypercalciuria may occur with sarcoidosis. The underlying mechanisms are not clear but increased sensitivity to vitamin D is one component. If unrecognized the calcium disturbances may lead to nephrocalcinosis, renal calculi and renal insufficiency.

Diagnosis and Investigations

1. CHEST RADIOGRAPH. Bilateral hilar lymph-gland enlargement is usually symmetrical with well defined outer borders. When pulmonary infiltration is present the shadows are about 5 mm in diameter and often predominantly in the mid zones with bilateral distribution. If fibrosis has occurred linear streaks radiating from the hila are usually visible.

2. KVEIM TEST. This is an intradermal injection of an homogenized suspension of human sarcoid spleen. The injection site is biopsied after six weeks. A positive result is obtained in 75–80 per cent of patients with sarcoidosis in the acute stages and is indicated by the presence of sarcoid granulomata. False positive results may be found in Crohn's disease and a number of other causes of chronic diarrhoea and lymph-node enlargement.

3. TISSUE BIOPSY. If readily accessible lymph nodes are present these should be excised and examined histologically. Biopsy of liver or mediastinal lymph nodes may also provide diagnostic tissue. Bronchial and alveolar tissue biopsies can be obtained through the fibreoptic bronchoscope, this has proved a very valuable means for establishing the diagnosis of sarcoidosis. If these methods fail to provide a diagnosis an open lung biopsy may occasionally be indicated.

4. TUBERCULIN TEST. About 60–75 per cent of patients with active sarcoidosis will give a negative result to one tuberculin unit in the Mantoux test.

5. OTHER TESTS. Hypercalcaemia is present in less than 5 per cent of patients and hypercalciuria in about 5–15 per cent. Rarely X-rays of the hands and feet may show lace-like thinning or longitudinal

streaks in the medulla of the phalanges of metacarpel and metatarsal bones.

6. LUNG FUNCTION CHANGES. With bilateral hilar lymphadenopathy alone it is uncommon to find abnormalities in lung function tests. Where radiological evidence of pulmonary infiltration is present or patients have symptoms of breathlessness the usual finding is a moderate restrictive ventilatory defect with reduction of static and dynamic lung volumes and gas transfer indices. Characteristically with sarcoidosis X-ray changes are more marked than the symptoms or physiological changes.

Course and Complications. Acute onset especially with erythema nodosum carries a good prognosis. Sixty to eighty per cent of patients with hilar lymphadenopathy alone may be expected to show complete radiographic clearing within one year and a further 10 per cent within a second year from diagnosis. Patients with pulmonary infiltration with or without hilar lymph-node enlargement have about a 50 per cent chance of spontaneous improvement within one year but if infiltration persists for more than two years, spontaneous remission is unlikely. In about half the patients with diffuse infiltration which persists this may remain static or progress very slowly to pulmonary fibrosis and breathlessness after five to ten years. The remaining patients with pulmonary infiltrates rapidly develop massive fibrosis with steady deterioration.

Treatment. Fever and arthralgia with hilar lymphadenopathy should be controlled by anti-inflammatory agents such as salicylates, phenylbutazone or indomethacin. *Indications for corticosteroid treatment* include eye involvement, hypercalcaemia, progressive pulmonary disease accompanied by breathlessness, and involvement of cardiovascular or nervous systems. Where indicated, treatment with prednisolone should be started at a dose of 30 or 40 mg daily; once a satisfactory response has been obtained this dose should be gradually reduced to a level which maintains the remission. If corticosteroids are contraindicated chloroquine has been found to suppress skin lesions and pulmonary infiltration but serious side effects limit its value.

EXTRINSIC ALLERGIC ALVEOLITIS

This group of diseases, due to hypersensitivity reactions to inhaled organic dusts mediated by precipitin antibody-antigen reactions (Gell and Coombs Type III). The commonest in the UK are farmer's lung and bird fancier's lung but other examples include pituitary snuff taker's lung, mushroom worker's lung, malt worker's lung, paprika splitter's lung and maple-bark splitter's lung, bagassosis (sugar cane handling).

Pathological Features. In acute episodes the alveoli are stuffed with desquamated cells, in more chronic cases these appearances are combined with alveolar wall fibrosis, the mixture varying from one region to another within the lung. Granuloma formation is common.

Clinical Features. During acute episodes symptoms occur 8–12 hours after exposure and consist of fever (39–40°C), chest tightness, muscle aches and pains, breathlessness with tachypnoea and unproductive cough. Malaise and headache may also be present. On examination of the chest, fine wheezes and crackles may be audible. The onset is more often insidious and at presentation breathlessness on exertion is marked, usually accompanied by cyanosis and finger clubbing.

Radiological Features. In the acute episode fine 'ground-glass' shadowing throughout the lungs may be present on chest X-ray. With chronic disease, fibrotic changes are particularly marked in the upper zones, with honeycombing in advanced disease.

Diagnosis. Usually made from a typical history of exposure and symptoms supported by the demonstration of specific serum precipitins.

Treatment. Removal from exposure to the antigen is vital. Steroids may be helpful in acute or subacute cases but have little effect with advanced fibrosis.

DIFFUSE FIBROSIS FROM DRUGS AND CHEMICALS

Busulphan may cause diffuse pneumonitis leading to widespread fibrosis. Occasionally stopping treatment may bring about resolution. *Bleomycin* causes an acute pulmonary reaction with exudates followed by diffuse fibrosis. With *nitrofurantoin* an acute exudative reaction may occur and insidious diffuse pulmonary fibrosis may result from long standing use of the drug. *Methysergide*, used for the treatment of migraine, has been known to cause pleural fibrosis and nodular lung fibrosis. *Hexamethonium* for the treatment of hypertension has been reported to cause widespread pulmonary fibrosis but differentiation of this from the results of longstanding left ventricular failure secondary to hypertensive heart disease is often difficult. The weedkiller *paraquat* causes an acute exudative desquamative reaction within the alveoli, followed by widespread fibrotic changes. Fatal poisoning may occur within 10–21 days from ingestion of very small quantities of the agricultural concentrate grammoxone. At least half the fatalities have been caused by intentional self-poisoning.

CRYPTOGENIC FIBROSING ALVEOLITIS

First described by Hamman and Rich as 'acute, widespread pulmonary shadows with severe breathlessness and death within a few months', is now recognized as a rare disorder with widespread desquamation of large numbers of cells within the alveolar spaces. The subacute or chronic form of the disease is much commoner and presents with insidious breathlessness, sometimes with unproductive cough, breathlessness at rest with profound hypoxia, right ventricular hypertrophy and right heart failure. Finger clubbing is present in 60–90 per cent of patients at presentation. The classic physical sign is widespread inspiratory crackles at the lung bases.

Lung Function Tests. There is usually a restrictive ventilatory defect with reduction of all lung volumes with reduced gas transfer. Profound arterial desaturation with exercise occurs with advanced disease.

Radiological Changes. The acute illness may present with 'ground-glass' or widespread mottled shadowing on chest X-ray. In chronic cases the shadows are mainly at the bases and may progress to honeycombing.

Associated Diseases. Polyarthritis is common and 30–50 per cent of patients have a positive rheumatoid serology while 10 per cent show features of clinical rheumatoid arthritis. Associations with chronic active hepatitis, renal tubular acidosis, dermatomyositis and a number of other disorders have been reported.

Diagnosis. This can often be made on the basis of the clinical features and X-rays, in the absence of occupational factors. Lung biopsy can be helpful in establishing the diagnosis and in staging the progress of the disease. Thus if the changes present are mainly of the desquamative type it is more likely that a good response will occur with treatment. For this purpose it is usually necessary to resort to open lung biopsy.

Prognosis. Variable, but deterioration is more rapid than with most other fibrosing lung diseases.

Treatment. Acute episodes respond well to corticosteroids such as prednisolone 40–60 mg daily for up to three months. The response in chronic cases is disappointing. A number of attempts have been made to use immunosuppressive agents including azathioprine, cyclophosphamide and more recently antifibrotic agents including penicillamine and colchicine have been tried with conflicting results.

SYSTEMIC DISEASES ASSOCIATED WITH DIFFUSE PULMONARY FIBROSIS

Rheumatoid Arthritis. In addition to pleurisy, pleural effusions and isolated pulmonary nodules, diffuse pulmonary fibrosis has been recognized as an uncommon feature of rheumatoid disease. The lower zones are usually predominantly affected and the disease is slowly progressive.

Systemic Sclerosis. This rare condition may occasionally cause diffuse pulmonary fibrosis of which the clinical, X-ray and physiological features are indistinguishable from those of other causes of diffuse fibrosis. In addition inhalation pneumonia and lung abscess are common, due to oesophageal involvement by the disease.

Systemic Lupus Erythematosus. This disease may cause pleurisy, pleural effusions and patchy recurrent shadows on chest X-ray due to pneumonitis. Diffuse pulmonary fibrosis is another common manifestation of this disease presenting as breathlessness and physiological changes indistinguishable from other causes of diffuse pulmonary fibrosis. The result is a restrictive ventilatory defect with reduced gas transfer. On chest X-ray the lungs appear small and the disorder has sometimes been referred to as the 'disappearing lung syndrome'.

OTHER CAUSES OF DIFFUSE PULMONARY SHADOWS

Bronchiectasis. Presenting with basal crepitations, finger clubbing and irregular shadows on chest X-ray may sometimes be confused with diffuse pulmonary fibrosis from other causes. Important points of differentiation are the long history of cough, production of purulent sputum, signs of airways obstruction and relative preservation of gas transfer.

Lymphangitis Carcinomatosa. May present with progressive breathlessness, reduced gas transfer and widespread pulmonary shadows. Lung biopsy may be necessary to establish the diagnosis but sometimes it may be made on sputum cytology.

Secondary Metastatic Disease, especially from carcinoma of the prostate in men and carcinoma of the breast in women.

Multiple Pulmonary Emboli. These sometimes result in progressive breathlessness with basal shadows on chest X-ray. Careful attention to history and physical signs will usually enable the differentiation to be made from diffuse pulmonary fibrosis.

Pulmonary Infiltration with Eosinophilia. A number of possible causes include:

1. SIMPLE PULMONARY EOSINOPHILIA ('Loeffler's syndrome'). Transient pulmonary shadows with reticular or nodular appearances often associated with reactions to drugs, e.g. sulphonamides, gold and PAS. It may also be caused by intestinal parasites. These shadows are usually fleeting, lasting less than 3 or 4 weeks and are associated with a high blood eosinophilia.
2. TROPICAL EOSINOPHILIA with or without asthma. This is usually due to sensitivity to intestinal and other parasites. Filariasis is probably the commonest cause throughout the world.

3. POLYARTERITIS NODOSA. May rarely present with fleeting pulmonary shadows associated with weight loss, skin rashes, peripheral neuropathy and blood eosinophilia.

4. PULMONARY EOSINOPHILIA WITH ASTHMA. The majority of patients with asthma who develop isolated fleeting shadows have allergic bronchopulmonary aspergillosis with serum precipitins to *Aspergillus fumigatus*. Rarely the same reactions may be due to hypersensitivity to *Candida albicans*. Other cases are idiopathic. The acute illness is characterized by febrile symptoms with muscle aches and pains associated with irregular patchy shadows on chest X-ray and a blood eosinophilia. Untreated the disease may progress to irregular pulmonary fibrosis and proximal bronchiectasis due to the impaction of sputum plugs containing *Aspergillus fumigatus* and the associated inflammatory reaction. Treatment with systemic corticosteroids may be necessary for long periods to suppress the immunological reactions and prevent lung damage.

Chapter 17

OCCUPATIONAL LUNG DISEASES

Asthma; Byssinosis; Pulmonary Exudates; Granulomatous Reactions; Pneumoconioses.

Injury to the lungs occurring at work may be caused by inhalation of gases, fumes, vapours, dusts or micro-organisms. The site and degree of the lung reaction is determined by the physical and chemical properties of the substance inhaled, the intensity and duration of exposure, the presence of pre-existing lung disease and individual differences in susceptibility.

The type of injury sustained by inhalation of gases is in part dependent on their solubility. Thus sulphur dioxide which is readily soluble produces an acute exudative reaction while toluene di-isocyanate (TDI) is without immediate clinical effect so that affected individuals may be subjected to repeated exposure before symptoms are noticed. With inorganic dusts the reaction is influenced by the dosage and particle size of the material as well as its chemical or physical properties. Only those dusts with a particle size in the range $0\cdot5-3$ μm can penetrate to the alveoli, larger particles being deposited within the airways and rapidly removed by ciliary transport and coughing. Similarly, only fibres with a diameter less then 3 μm can penetrate beyond the terminal bronchioles. Dust particles which have penetrated beyond the ciliated epithelium are engulfed by alveolar macrophages and these may then be transported by the ciliary mechanism or pass into the perivascular lymphatic channels. What effects then follow depends both upon the quantity of dust inhaled and its physical and chemical properties. If the quantity inhaled overwhelms the clearance mechanisms of the lung dust-laden macrophages will accumulate. Inert substances such as iron, tin and carbon will have little injurious effect and although the accumulation of macrophages laden with these substances may produce dramatic radio-opacities on chest X-ray there is little or no fibrosis. Conversely silica or asbestos cause macrophage cytotoxicity with marked fibrotic reactions. In addition the fibrous dusts tend to drift towards the pleura leading to extensive pleural fibrosis.

OCCUPATIONAL ASTHMA

Although atopic individuals may develop hypersensitivity to substances inhaled at work (immediate IgE mediated, Gell and Coombs Type I hypersensitivity) the majority of cases of occupational asthma are non-atopic and in most instances the underlying mechanisms have not yet been fully evaluated. Occupational asthma is particularly common in laboratory staff working with experimental animals, notably rats, mice, rabbits and guinea-

131

pigs. In the case of asthma induced by rats it has been shown that affected individuals are sensitized by a protein excreted in the urine of male rats. As with many of the other forms of occupational asthma, although affected individuals are usually non-atopic, it seems likely that hypersensitization is the cause as only a minority of individuals exposed develop symptoms. There is usually a latent interval of weeks to years between first exposure and the onset of asthma and asthma can be induced in affected individuals by exposure to minute concentrations of the offending agent.

Other recognized causes of occupational asthma include the isocyanates TDI (toluene di-isocyanate) and MDI (di-isocyanato diphenyl methane) which are used in the production of polyurethane plastics, complex salts of platinum (chloroplatinates) in refinery workers, pine resin (colophony) used in multicore solders by electricians and assembly workers in the electronics industry and the proteolytic enzymes of *Bacillus subtilis* in biological washing powders. Asthma induced by detergent enzymes has only occurred in workers involved in the manufacture of these powders who have been found to have serum IgE antibodies to *B. subtilis* proteins; it does not occur in those using the powders for washing. Occupational asthma may also develop due to exposure to the wheat weevil *Sitophilus granarius*, gum arabic (Acacia senegal) in printing inks and hardwood or redwood dusts.

When searching for occupational factors in asthma a very careful history is necessary in order to make the diagnosis because the asthmatic reactions do not develop until several hours after exposure. An important point is that symptoms may remit at week-ends and on holidays. Final recognition of the causative agent may only be possible by challenge tests in which the patient is exposed to the suspected substance under carefully controlled conditions. Because severe airways obstruction can result from exposure to minute quantities of the offending substance these tests are best left to specialist units.

Clinical Features. No unique clinical features are usually noticeable in patients with occupational asthma and when seen at a routine consultation they may well be devoid of abnormal physical signs.

It is important to recognize occupational causes of asthma as this is one of the few occasions when asthma may be said to be cured if the individual is removed from exposure to the causative substance.

Treatment. Often the only satisfactory treatment may be a change of employment together with symptomatic measures to relieve airways obstruction. On occasions it may be necessary to resort to corticosteroids for control of severe asthma in affected patients.

BYSSINOSIS

This is a disorder arising in workers exposed to dusts associated with the processing of raw cotton, flax and hemp. The effects usually occur after several years of exposure and those individuals working in the earliest part of the processing of the raw materials are most often affected. It seems to be caused by a hypersensitivity reaction to a substance in the cotton bract which is a potent liberator of histamine. The disease is more common in non-smokers.

Clinical Features. The 'Monday feeling' with breathlessness and chest tightness first occurs only on return to work at the beginning of each week. Signs of airways obstruction are usually present when patients are breathless. At first the symptoms improve towards the end of the week but eventually breathlessness, cough and sputum develop and the condition is indistinguishable from chronic bronchitis.

Diagnosis. This is made on the basis of occupation, the timing of symptoms and signs of transient airways obstruction. There are no specific abnormalities visible on chest X-rays.

Treatment. The affected individual must avoid all further exposure to cotton bract and may be given symptomatic relief with a bronchodilator.

PULMONARY EXUDATES

EXTRINSIC ALLERGIC ALVEOLITIS

Many of the causes of extrinsic allergic alveolitis are connected with noxious agents encountered at work including farmer's lung, mushroom worker's lung, malt worker's lung, bagassosis etc. and as such are occupational lung diseases but this group is dealt with elsewhere (*see* Chapter 16).

PULMONARY OEDEMA

Many gases and fumes are capable of producing pulmonary oedema with damage to the respiratory epithelium and alveolar capillaries. Of particular importance are ozone, chlorine, ammonia, oxides of nitrogen, fumes of beryllium, cadmium, magnesium, vanadium and tungsten. Exposure may occur accidentally but certain occupations are particularly at risk. There is commonly a latent interval of 12 hours or more between exposure and the onset of pulmonary oedema. One exception is sulphur dioxide which because of its marked solubility produces acute symptoms immediately.

WELDING

Welders may be exposed to fumes of zinc, copper, vanadium and fluorine as well as oxides of nitrogen released during electric arc and oxyacetylene welding if poor ventilation in confined spaces prevents dispersion of these gases and fumes.

SILO WORKERS

Oxides of nitrogen may form from nitrous oxide produced from plant nitrates and collect together with ammonia and carbon dioxide in confined spaces at the top of agricultural silos. When inhaled by workers entering the top of these towers they may cause acute pulmonary oedema. Silo workers occasionally develop extrinsic allergic alveolitis to *Micropolyspora faeni* (mouldy hay) and *Sitophilus granarius* (wheat weevil).

MINING ˙

Very occasionally exposure to toxic concentrations of oxides of nitrogen from shot blasting may develop if ventilation is poor.

Clinical Features. Exposure to ammonia, chlorine and bromine usually causes immediate symptoms of irritation of the trachea and bronchi. Pulmonary oedema caused by exposure to oxides of nitrogen and ozone may be delayed for up to 24 hours and is heralded by symptoms of restlessness, fatigue, anxiety, cough, frothy sputum with or without blood staining, breathlessness and shallow respirations, with cyanosis in severe cases. Death occasionally occurs from asphyxia but the majority recover completely. Some individuals exposed to oxides of nitrogen get recurrent pulmonary oedema and develop an obliterative bronchiolitis.

Radiological Features. The chest X-ray may show the typical 'bat's wing' distribution of ill-defined patchy shadowing of pulmonary oedema.

Treatment. This consists of warmth, rest and oxygen therapy with tracheal aspiration and artificial ventilation if the ventilatory impairment progresses. Fluid replacement may be necessary to correct haemoconcentration where this occurs, with intravenous hydrocorticone followed by prednisolone in severe cases.

METAL FUME FEVER

Brazing with solders containing zinc or burning or welding zinc-plated metals in enclosed spaces may give rise to symptoms of 'metal fume fever'. Fumes of cadmium, magnesium, vanadium, zinc and tungsten are less toxic.

Clinical Features. Symptoms and signs are delayed for several hours and consist of fever, generalized muscular aches and severe chest pain, vomiting and diarrhoea. Heavy exposure may cause fatal haemorrhagic pulmonary oedema, toxic hepatitis and rarely renal cortical necrosis. In less severe cases complete recovery may occur. Chronic exposure to low concentrations of cadmium dust may cause proteinuria and renal tubular defects.

Treatment. This is as for toxic gases but in addition cautious use of the chelating agent calcium EDTA may be useful.

GRANULOMATOUS REACTIONS.

Pulmonary granulomas are a feature of a number of lung reactions related to occupation. *Talc granulomas:* exposure to talc may cause multiple small granulomas containing talc crystals.

Radiological Features. Multiple small opacities similar to miliary tuberculosis or sarcoidosis.

Clinical Features. It may be symptomless or there may be mild effort dyspnoea with a restrictive ventilatory defect and moderate impairment of gas transfer.

Treatment. If symptoms warrant their use, corticosteroids may cause some improvement by suppressing the granulomas.

BERYLLIUM DISEASE

Beryllium is widely used in the aerospace industries but strict controls have reduced the risks of occupational exposure to occasional accidents. It may be inhaled in the form of dust or fumes in metallurgical industries, as oxides used in the manufacture of ceramics and as salts in laboratories. The acute disease produces pulmonary oedema but the chronic form is characterized by the formation of multiple sarcoid-like granulomas with interstitial fibrosis. This develops in a very small proportion of those exposed.

Clinical Features
ACUTE EXPOSURE. Acute massive exposure gives rise to severe pulmonary oedema after a delay of 48–72 hours. The mortality is high. Lesser exposure leads to a slowly developing pneumonitis which may resolve if re-exposure is prevented. The symptoms are breathlessness and cyanosis.

Radiological Features. Widespread 'ground-glass' shadowing.
CHRONIC DISEASE. This may begin insidiously or follow repeated acute episodes. Although it resembles sarcoidosis there are striking differences. Erythema nodosum, lupus pernio, bone changes and uveitis do not occur with beryllium disease and the fibrosis is always progressive. The Kveim test is negative and tuberculin reactivity is unaltered.

Clinical Features. Are those of diffuse interstitial fibrosis with progressive dyspnoea and arterial desaturation. Death from right heart failure is common.

Radiological Features. Are of a non-specific diffuse fibrosis.

Treatment. Corticosteroids may prevent the progression of the disease.

PNEUMOCONIOSES

At the present time dust-related lung changes or the pneumoconioses are numerically the most important form of occupational lung disease in the UK.

BENIGN NON-FIBROTIC PNEUMOCONIOSES

These are recognized by the presence of multiple small dense opacities on chest X-ray due to perivascular collections of dust with increase in reticulin fibres but no collagen changes. Lung function is unchanged and there are no symptoms.

SIDEROSIS

This is the commonest benign pneumonociosis, caused by iron dust in the mining and processing of iron ore and steel and the manufacture of emery abrasives. Welders may also be affected by inhalation of fumes of oxides of iron.

STANNOSIS

Caused by inhalation of tin dust during the processing of the crude ore and inhalation of tin oxide fumes in smelting is rare as are other benign pneumoconioses caused by barium sulphate, antimony and chromite dusts.

FIBROTIC PNEUMOCONIOSES

COAL WORKER'S PNEUMOCONIOSIS

This is the commonest occupational lung disease in Britain, the prevalence in coal workers being about 10 per cent but it was a much greater problem until more rigorous dust suppression was introduced about 20 years ago. Clinically it is helpful to distinguish simple pneumoconiosis and progressive massive fibrosis.

SIMPLE PNEUMOCONIOSIS

The earliest lesions are small, discrete aggregates of coal dust up to 4 mm in diameter around alveoli with some increase in reticulin fibres. There may be an associated non-destructive centrilobular emphysema in the vicinity of the dust nodules. This may not be a specific feature of pneumoconiosis, but rather an effect of the coal dust accentuating emphysema which has developed from other causes such as cigarette-smoking.

Clinical Features. There are no specific symptoms or signs of simple pneumoconiosis and there is no detectable impairment of lung function. In patients with symptoms and X-ray changes of simple pneumoconiosis care should be taken to exclude the coexistence of chronic bronchitis, asthma or heart failure. At present it is uncertain whether simple pneumoconiosis alone causes airway narrowing.

Radiological Features. The characteristic appearances are of fine nodular shadows mainly affecting the upper halves of the lung fields. Through the International Labour Office (ILO) a system of classification has been developed for scoring the profusion and the size of the individual shadows. These are mainly of use for epidemiological studies in relating the size of the shadows to the quantity of dust in the lungs and the degree of dust exposure.

Treatment. Simple pneumoconiosis requires no specific treatment.

PROGRESSIVE MASSIVE FIBROSIS (PMF)

This form of pneumoconiosis develops in a minority of coal workers and very similar forms are seen in workers in the synthetic graphite and carbon black industries. Large masses of coal dust and irregular hyalinized collagen form in the upper zones and this progresses to necrosis and cavitation which may continue or develop after exposure has ceased. The tendency to develop PMF seems to be related to the degree of dust exposure. Tuberculosis and silica in the coal have been excluded as causes of PMF which seems likely to be the result of an abnormal immunological susceptibility in affected individuals.

Radiological Features. The ILO classification divides the shadows into 3 classes, A, B and C in ascending order of severity as represented by the area covered on chest X-rays.

Clinical Features. Complicated pneumoconiosis may be a cause of severe disability. Patients with extensive shadowing are usually breathless but some patients with PMF may be symptomless. Sometimes the necrotic fibrous tissue may be discharged into a bronchus and coughed up. The symptoms depend on the site of the lesions. If the masses develop in the mid zones and extend to involve the pulmonary arteries severe pulmonary hypertension with cor pulmonale may develop. Again involvement of large bronchi in the fibrotic process leads to signs and symptoms of airways obstruction.

Lung Function Features. There is often a restrictive ventilatory defect with reduced gas transfer. However, if extensive fibrosis involves the airways there will be evidence of airways obstruction.

Treatment. There is no effective treatment to prevent extension of PMF once established.

RHEUMATOID COAL PNEUMOCONIOSIS (CAPLAN'S SYNDROME)

Some coal workers may develop multiple nodules visible on chest X-ray as opacities 1–2 cm in diameter. These develop more rapidly than in PMF and are usually associated with minimal shadowing of pneumoconiosis. Histologically, these nodules resemble subcutaneous rheumatoid nodules. Affected individuals are seropositive for rheumatoid factor but the clinical signs of rheumatoid arthritis are often minimal and the lung nodules may sometimes predate the onset of arthritis. Pleural effusions may occasionally occur in affected individuals.

SILICOSIS

Silicosis, once a common disorder, occurs less often now due to better dust control. It results from inhalation of silica dust from quartz and flint and is a hazard in quarrying, mining and sandblasting industries and in foundries where sand moulds and refractory linings to kilns are used. Sand blasting has been banned in the UK for 20 years but is still permitted in the USA. The principal lesion is a grey nodule 2–5 mm in diameter formed of concentric layers of collagen. There is no associated emphysema.

Radiological Features. The nodules appear as discrete opacities mainly in the upper zones on chest X-ray and may increase in size with time and become conglomerate resembling the opacities seen in PMF. 'Eggshell' calcification may develop at the periphery of hilar lymph nodes.

Clinical Features. Once exposure has resulted in the appearance of visible X-ray changes the disease is usually progressive. Simple nodular silicosis is symptomless but a troublesome cough develops as the nodules increase in size. Extensive lung damage and fibrosis from conglomerate silicosis may lead to severe breathlessness with a restrictive ventilatory defect and impaired gas transfer. Silicosis predisposes to pulmonary tuberculosis.

ASBESTOSIS

Chief sources of exposure have been in asbestos cement and textile factories, insulation work and spraying in buildings and ships. Asbestos exposure may cause pulmonary fibrosis, pleural fibrosis and calcification, carcinoma of the bronchus and pleural mesothelioma. Three types of asbestos, chrysotile (white), crocidolite (blue) and amosite (brown), have been widely used; all may cause pulmonary fibrosis but the risks of mesothelioma are greater with crocidolite than with the other forms.

Pulmonary fibrosis apart from asbestos usually follows heavy industrial exposure over a period of many years and is most marked in the lower zones and pleural thickening with calcification is common. Many affected individuals go on to develop *bronchial carcinoma* and a synergistic oncogenic effect with cigarette smoke may occur. Asbestos probably acts as a co-carcinogen increasing the risk of bronchial carcinoma in cigarette smokers. *Mesothelioma* is commonest in individuals who have heavy occupational exposure to asbestos but only light exposure is necessary and cases have been recorded in individuals living near to asbestos works who have not had occupational exposure. The tumour develops 30–40 years after exposure.

Asbestos Bodies: The presence of asbestos fibres coated in a gold-coloured iron and protein covering as asbestos bodies in the sputum indicates past exposure to asbestos but is not diagnostic of asbestosis.

Clinical Features. Except where changes on chest X-ray lead to medical examination of an asymptomatic individual, most patients with asbestosis present with breathlessness on effort. As the disease progresses characteristic changes in lung function occur with restriction of ventilatory capacity and total lung volume and reduced gas transfer. Most patients develop finger clubbing and cyanosis and the characteristic physical sign of late inspiratory crackles may be heard at the lung bases.

Radiological Features. Diffuse interstitial fibrosis shows as shadowing, most marked in the lower zones, sometimes with a honeycomb pattern. Fibrosis of the parietal pleura with irregular calcification is common.

MALIGNANT MESOTHELIOMA

This may develop in the pleura or peritoneum after brief exposure to asbestos, crocidolite is the usual form involved. The histological appearances show features resembling adenocarcinoma as well as other more frankly sarcomatous changes.

Clinical Features. The commonest clinical presentation is as a painful pleural effusion. Although distant metastases are usually found at post-mortem they are rarely clinically apparent during life.

Treatment. Radiotherapy, cytotoxic agents and surgery are ineffective. Whenever possible the diagnosis should be established without operation to delay extension of the growth through the chest wall.

Chapter 18

DRUGS AND THE LUNGS

Antibiotics; Bronchodilators; Corticosteroids. Adverse reactions to drugs including: Asthma; Pulmonary Eosinophilia; Pulmonary Fibrosis; Systemic Lupus Erythematosus; Polyarteritis Nodosa; Thrombo-embolic Disease; Lipoid Pneumonia; Oxygen Toxicity.

ANTIBIOTICS FOR PULMONARY INFECTIONS (*see Table* 4, p. 99)

General principles to be considered:
1. Is an antibiotic necessary?
2. Which drug and what dose is appropriate?
3. The sensitivities of the organism involved.
4. Potential hypersensitivity of the patient.
5. Renal and hepatic function should be assessed, especially if drugs such as streptomycin are to be given.

General Principles
1. Wherever possible choose bactericidal rather than bacteriostatic drugs, especially for severe infections and for immunodeficient patients.
2. Benzylpenicillin is the antibiotic of choice for susceptible organisms.
3. Drug combinations should be chosen to prevent resistance developing, e.g. staphylococci easily develop resistance to erythromycin.
4. Possible initial drug resistance, e.g. many strains of *H. influenzae* are resistant to co-trimoxazole.
5. Cross-resistance, e.g. if an organism is resistant to cloxacillin it will also be resistant to methicillin and cephaloridine.

Conditions where Antibiotic Treatment is indicated. Include pneumonia, acute bronchitis, exacerbartions of chronic bronchitis, acute asthma with purulent sputum, exacerbations of bronchiectasis, lung abscess, empyema.

Investigations. Sputum specimens should be obtained before giving an antibiotic and examined by Gram stain, culture and sensitivities, including anaerobes. Blood cultures may be helpful, especially in pneumonia.

Suggestions for Choice of Antibiotic
1. Pneumonia: usually penicillin and ampicillin are suitable, amoxycillin may come to replace ampicillin.
2. Exacerbations of chronic bronchitis: are usually caused by *S. pneumoniae* or *H. influenzae*. Ampicillin or amoxycillin are the drugs of choice.
3. *S. aureus* infections should be treated with cloxacillin or methicillin as these are effective against penicillinase-producing staphylococci.

For *patients with histories of hypersensitivity* such as rashes or fevers following penicillins, choose a tetracycline, co-trimoxazole or erythromycin.

BRONCHODILATOR TREATMENT

For the relief of airways obstruction in asthma and chronic bronchitis these drugs are available as oral, aerosol and parenteral preparations.

1. Oral Preparations. These are useful for maintenance treatment. Wherever possible avoid combination preparations which usually contain small quantities of barbiturates and ineffective doses of bronchodilators. The main groups available include ephedrine, theophyllines, and the beta-sympathomimetic agents. Ephedrine is often effective in children but may cause urinary retention in elderly men. The theophylline group often cause nausea and abdominal discomfort, this may be lessened by the use of one of the slowly released preparations such as phyllocontin (amino-phylline). The sympathomimetic agents including orciprenaline, salbutamol, terbutaline, rimiterol and fenoterol are effective bronchodilators but commonly cause peripheral muscle tremor when given by mouth. There are theoretical grounds for combining a theophylline oral agent with a sympathomimetic aerosol as these may have different sites of action on airways.

2. Aerosol Preparations. These give standard metered doses of broncho-dilator both as pressurized wet aerosols and more recently as dry powder aerosols. By inhalation a more rapid onset of action is achieved but many patients find it difficult to master the technique of inhaling from pressurized aerosols. Aerosols may be ineffective in the presence of severe airways obstruction. Sympathomimetic agents available as aerosols include isoprenaline which, wherever possible, should be avoided because of its lack of selectivity and tendency to cause tachycardias; orciprenaline, salbutamol, rimiterol, terbutaline and fenoterol.

OTHER FORMS OF AEROSOL THERAPY. The drugs listed above may all be inhaled as a wet aerosol from a Wright's nebulizer or by intermittent positive-pressure breathing equipment. The greater effectiveness of this method for producing bronchodilatation may purely reflect the large doses given by this route.

3. Parenteral Treatment. *Aminophylline* should be given by continuous infusion, e.g. 500 mg 8-hourly in 5 per cent dextrose or less advisedly as a slow intravenous injection over 15–30 minutes. A check should be kept of sweating, faintness, increasing tachycardia or signs of cerebral irritation. *Salbutamol* is available for intravenous infusion. *Terbutaline* is available for subcutaneous injection. *Adrenaline* is a very effective bronchodilator when given by subcutaneous injection which may be painful.

CORTICOSTEROID TREATMENT

Drugs with glucocorticoid actions are widely used in the treatment of lung diseases, e.g.

1. For the relief of airways obstruction in asthma.
2. Treatment of pulmonary eosinophilia.
3. For allergic alveolitis and cryptogenic fibrosing alveolitis.
4. Sarcoidosis with pulmonary infiltration where respiratory symptoms are prominent.
5. For a variety of less common disorders including collagen diseases, eosinophilic granuloma etc.

All patients on corticosteroid therapy should carry a steroid identification card.

Asthma. Because of the numerous side effects wherever possible corticosteroids should be administered by topical application as aerosols. At present two are available, beclomethasone dipropionate and betamethasone valerate. Both have marked topical activity and in the doses recommended do not produce hypothalamo-pituitary-adrenal suppression. For chronic asthma corticosteroid treatment may be initiated with these preparations, or, alternatively, they may be used to reduce the dose of systemic corticosteroids already in use for control of asthma. Some patients develop oropharyngeal candidiasis while using steroid aerosols but treatment need not be stopped as this infection usually responds to amphotericin B lozenges. For maintenance treatment with systemic corticosteroids there seem to be no good reasons for choosing drugs other than prednisolone. For patients with gastrointestinal symptoms the enteric-coated form may be prescribed. Where possible treatment should be given on an alternate-day basis as this minimizes the likelihood of side effects and hypothalamo-pituitary-adrenal suppression.

Childhood Asthma. For most children with asthma severe enough to require corticosteroids for maintenance treatment this can usually be given by aerosol. Where parenteral corticosteroid therapy proves essential it has been claimed that the use of injections of corticotrophin (ACTH) or tetracosactrin depot (Synacthen) may lead to less growth retardation and less marked effects upon the hypothalamo-pituitary-adrenal axis than oral steroid therapy.

ADVERSE LUNG REACTIONS TO DRUGS

Up to 5 per cent of all hospital admissions are caused by adverse reactions to drugs and in hospital 10—15 per cent of patients may suffer such reactions and about 3 per cent of hospital deaths are related to drug toxicity. Lung disease may result from drugs which have been inhaled, ingested or injected. In many instances the mechanism of adverse lung reactions is not understood but a number of general principles should be borne in mind.

1. DOSAGE. The incidence of side effects tends to increase with increasing size of dose but hypersensitivity reactions are not dose-related.

2. ALTERED METABOLISM OR EXCRETION. Hepatic or renal insufficiency may result in increased plasma concentration of drugs and toxic levels may be reached with conventional doses. The very young and old are particularly susceptible.

3. GENETIC FACTORS. As yet no lung reaction to drugs has been clearly associated with genetic predisposition.

4. DRUG INTERACTIONS
   a. *Interference* may occur by altered responsiveness at receptor sites without increase in concentration.
   b. *Alteration of drug concentration*, e.g. barbiturates may increase liver enzyme function necessitating larger doses of corticosteroids as these are then more rapidly metabolized.
   c. *Altered immunity:* Corticosteroids and immunosuppressive agents may render patients more susceptible to infections.
   d. *Hypersensitivity Reactions:* A number of different types including pulmonary eosinophilia, polyarteritis nodosa, systemic lupus erythematosus and pulmonary fibrosis may result from adverse reactions to drugs.

5. TREATMENT HISTORY. Details of previous adverse reactions to drugs including any history of anaphylaxis, skin rashes or wheezing should be sought. Details of current treatment should be recorded. The presence of hepatic and renal disease should be excluded. A history of atopy in the patient or his family should also be noted.

Drug-induced Asthma. Asthma may be provoked by drugs in several ways:

1. SIMPLE IRRITATION. For example inhalation of sodium cromoglycate powder (Intal) may induce reflex airways obstruction.

2. DIRECT PHARMACOLOGICAL ACTION. Drugs which block beta-sympathomimetic nerve receptors such as propranolol or oxprenolol may cause increased airways obstruction in patients with asthma by effects at beta-2-receptors. Metoprolol seems less likely to do this as it is more selective.

3. INDIRECT PHARMACOLOGICAL ACTION. Acetylsalicylic acid (aspirin) may provoke asthma especially in patients with late-onset asthma and nasal polyposis. This reaction comes on between half-an-hour and two hours after ingestion of the drug. Cross-sensitivity with other non-steroidal anti-inflammatory agents including indomethacin, and ibuprofen has been noted. This effect is thought to be mediated through alterations in the balance of E and F series prostaglandins.

4. PARADOXICAL EFFECT OF BRONCHODILATORS. It is claimed that some patients with extrinsic allergic asthma may show a paradoxical airway narrowing after inhalation of isoprenaline.

5. HYPERSENSITIVITY ASTHMA. Allergic reactions causing airways obstruction, urticaria and occasionally anaphylactic shock have been recorded with a wide variety of drugs, such as antibiotics including penicillins, streptomycin, tetracycline, erythromycin, neomycin and mono-amine oxidase inhibitors, local anaesthetics and vaccines. Most of these reactions are probably mediated by IgE antibodies in type I immediate hypersensitivity reactions and occasionally more delayed reactions mediated by IgG antibodies may occur.

Pulmonary Eosinophilia. Acute exudative lung reactions with blood and pulmonary eosinophilia have been recorded to a wide variety of drugs, including aspirin, furazolidone, imipramine, isoniazid, methenycin, methotrexate, nitrofurantoin, PAS, penicillin, streptomycin and sulphonamides.

Clinical Features: The onset is acute with breathlessness audible throughout the chest.

The *chest X-ray* shows diffuse irregular shadowing sometimes with small pleural effusions. Blood and sputum eosinophilia are usually present.

Lung function tests in the acute phase show reduction of lung volume and carbon monoxide transfer factor with hypoxaemia and hypocapnia.

Treatment: Most cases recover spontaneously if the drug is discontinued but sometimes corticosteroids may be necessary.

Polyarteritis Nodosa. Many drugs have been reported to cause variants of polyarteritis nodosa with an allergic granulomatous angiitis affecting small veins and arteries of the lungs. There may be eosinophilic infiltration leading to the formation of giant-cell granulomas.

Amongst the drugs implicated are the sulphonamides, iodides, penicillins, arsenicals, mercurials, gold salts and phenothiazines.

Systemic Lupus Erythematosus (SLE). In about 20 per cent of patients with SLE the onset may be linked to drugs, those most often incriminated are hydrallazine, phenytoin, procainamide, and isoniazid but a large number of others including streptomycin, antihypertensive agents, practolol and other beta-blocking drugs and antibacterial agents including penicillins and sulphonamides may also induce this response.

Clinical manifestation of lung involvement include:

1. PLEURISY WITH PLEURAL EFFUSIONS. Usually bilateral, often accompanied by pericarditis and fever.

2. FEBRILE EPISODES. With cough, breathlessness, pleurisy and pneumonitis, sometimes progressing to pulmonary oedema or pulmonary infarction.

3. PROGRESSIVE BREATHLESSNESS. With reduced chest expansion, elevation of the diaphragms ('the disappearing lung syndrome').

Drug-induced SLE shows certain features which are atypical compared with the characteristic disease:

1. It is commoner in men.
2. The lungs are much more frequently involved.
3. The kidneys are usually spared.
4. The anti-DNA antibodies are against single-strand denatured DNA not double-strand native DNA.
5. Serum complement levels are unchanged.

Drug-induced SLE may be irreversible but usually improves on withdrawing the drug.

Pulmonary Fibrosis. A number of drugs have been shown to produce intra-alveolar exudates progressing to chronic fibrosis. They include: cytotoxic agents such as bleomycin, busulphan, chlorambucil, cyclophosphamide, methotrexate and vincristine. Ganglion-blocking antihypertensive agents including hexamethonium, pentolinium and mecamylamine. Antibacterial agents, nitrofurantoin and sulphasalazine may produce infiltrates but probably do not progress to fibrosis. Extrinsic allergic alveolitis progressing to pulmonary fibrosis may be caused by inhalation of pituitary snuff. The acute reaction is characterized by symptoms of pulmonary oedema. At the chronic stage widespread crepitations are present and the chest X-ray shows extensive nodular patchy shadows. Lung function tests show the characteristic combination of a restrictive ventilatory defect with reduced gas transfer.

Thrombo-embolic Disease affecting the Lungs. Oral contraceptives containing high doses of oestrogens have been shown to cause acute and chronic pulmonary embolic disease but the new combined progestogen-oestrogen preparations with an oestrogen content below 50 mg seem to be safer.

Lipoid Pneumonia and Oil Embolism. Chronic ingestion of liquid paraffin, oily medicines such as cod liver oil and rarely the oil-based contrast media used for bronchography may cause granulomatous lung reactions especially at the bases. These may progress to cause diffuse pulmonary fibrosis or a localized solid mass. Rarely, lung reactions may occur to lymphangiographic contrast media.

Oxygen-induced Lung Disease. Prolonged use of high inspired oxygen concentrations (greater than 60 per cent) may result in widespread lung changes. These include:

1. Patchy atelectasis caused by replacement of alveolar nitrogen by oxygen with absorption collapse of alveoli.
2. An exudative reaction with alveolar haemorrhage, fibrinous exudate and hyaline membrane formation.
3. Irreversible fibrosis with hyperplasia of the alveolar epithelium.

Opportunist Infections. Treatment with corticosteroids and immuno-suppressive drugs may predispose to infection with opportunist organisms (*see* Chapter 15).

Chapter 19

MALIGNANT DISEASES AND BENIGN TUMOURS OF THE LUNGS

Bronchial Carcinoma; Bronchial Adenoma; Hamartoma; Malignant Invasion of the Lungs; Mesothelioma.

The lungs are a common site of primary and metastatic malignant disease, benign tumours being much less common.

CARCINOMA OF THE BRONCHUS

Incidence and Epidemiology. Throughout the civilized world there has been a dramatic increase in the incidence of carcinoma of the bronchus in the last 50 years. In Britain it is now the commonest primary neoplasm in men and in recent years there has been a sharp increase in its incidence in women. In England and Wales, the mortality rate in men is about 250 per 100 000 and in women 100 per 100 000. This is a disease of middle and old age, about half the deaths occurring before the age of 65.

Aetiology. Three major factors have been recognized: cigarette smoking, atmospheric pollution, industrial hazards.

SMOKING. The risk of developing bronchial carcinoma is directly related to the daily consumption of cigarettes, so that in men who smoke more than 25 cigarettes a day the risk of developing lung cancer is 20 times greater than for non-smokers. Pipe and cigar smokers show a risk 2 or 3 times greater than non-smokers. Giving up smoking helps, the excess mortality in cigarette smokers is halved 5 years after stopping smoking. The carcinogens in tobacco smoke include polycyclic aromatic hydrocarbons, phenols, fatty acid esters and free fatty acids. Of the various types of lung cancer only adenocarcinoma and alveolar-cell carcinoma are not directly caused by smoking and the incidence of the commonest types, squamous- and oat-cell is directly related to smoking habits.

ATMOSPHERIC POLLUTION. There is an excess mortality of about 2 to 1 in urban compared to rural populations for bronchial carcinoma in both smokers and non-smokers.

INDUSTRIAL HAZARDS. Asbestos is the most widespread and dangerous industrial cause of lung cancer. Increased risk has also been recognized in uranium miners, and with exposure to chromates, nickel, arsenic and radioactive gases.

Pathology. Four main histological types of bronchial carcinoma are recognized:

Squamous-cell carcinoma accounting for 40—55 per cent of the total.

Anaplastic small-cell or oat-cell, 25—35 per cent.

Undifferentiated large cell, 10—20 per cent.

Adenocarcinoma, 4—10 per cent.

Alveolar-cell carcinoma, 1 per cent or less.

Squamous- and oat-cell carcinoma are about 4 times commoner in men than women but adenocarcinoma is only twice as common in men. Half or more of all bronchial carcinomas arise in the segmental or more proximal bronchi. Squamous- and oat-cell carcinomas tend to arise from the central bronchi while adenocarcinomas tend to be more peripheral in site. Tumours may spread by direct invasion of the lung, chest wall, mediastinal structures and by metastasis to hilar and mediastinal lymph nodes. Bloodborne metastasis is common to the liver, adrenal glands, bones and brain. Symptoms may arise through local spread with bronchial irritation, ulceration and obstruction. Secondary pneumonia or lung abscess may occur due to infection distal to the tumour. Other symptoms and signs may arise as a result of metastases or non-metastatic extrapulmonary manifestations.

Clinical Features

1. CHEST SYMPTOMS. *Cough* is common and often ignored or passed off as chronic bronchitis. *Breathlessness* is common but rarely disabling unless caused by obstruction of a major bronchus, lymphangitis carcinomatosa or a large pleural effusion. *Haemoptysis,* frequently the first symptom, occurs in more than half the patients but massive haemorrhage is rare. *Chest pain,* presenting as three main types, a persistent dull aching; pleuritic due to secondary pneumonia or from malignant invasion of the pleura, and thirdly, chest wall pain from local invasion of the ribs and intercostal nerves by tumour. *Hoarseness* is common, usually due to left recurrent laryngeal nerve palsy from hilar extension of the tumour or enlargement of mediastinal lymph glands. Three common clinical presentations of bronchial carcinoma should be recognized, especially in middle-aged smokers.

   a. *Pneumonia.* Commonly the first manifestation. Failure to clear with antibiotic treatment or the recurrence of a pneumonia in the same segment or lobe should suggest an underlying tumour.

   b. *Lung Abscess.* Frequent presentation of carcinoma of the bronchus.

   c. *Recurrent Chest Infections.* In a previously healthy cigarette smoker should always raise the suspicion of a slowly enlarging tumour.

   General Symptoms. About 10—15 per cent of patients present with non-specific symptoms of fever, weight loss, weakness, tiredness and anorexia. Severe weight loss is a late sign of carcinoma of the bronchus. Clubbing of the fingers, especially of rapid onset, is suggestive of bronchial neoplasm but only occurs in about 15 per cent of patients. It is rare with adenocarcinoma and oat-cell tumours.

Chest Signs. Commonly there are no specific physical signs present although evidence of collapse or consolidation of a segment or lobe of the lung or of a pleural effusion may be present. *Pleural effusions* secondary to infection distal to a carcinoma are common, more rarely direct invasion of the pleura by tumour may cause a bloodstained effusion which reaccumulates rapidly after aspiration. Rarely a localized low-pitched wheeze due to partial obstruction of a bronchus may be audible.

2. NERVE INVOLVEMENT. Left recurrent laryngeal nerve palsy causing hoarseness or paralysis of a hemidiaphragm by phrenic nerve involvement is common. Horner's syndrome resulting from invasion of the cervical sympathetic trunk by apical tumours causes ptosis, meiosis, enophthalmos and loss of sweating on the affected half of the face. Brachial plexus involvement causes pain, weakness and paraesthesiae in the arm and hand.

3. RIB EROSION. Will cause chest wall pain with localized tenderness.

4. SUPERIOR VENA CAVAL OBSTRUCTION. This is common with tumours of the right upper lobe or with mediastinal masses. Typical features are swelling, oedema and cyanosis of the face and upper limbs with non-pulsatile distension of the veins.

5. PERICARDIAL INVOLVEMENT. Uncommon but may cause cardiac arrhythmias or rarely tamponade.

6. OESOPHAGEAL OBSTRUCTION. Dysphagia from invasion of the oesophagus occurs in a minority of patients.

7. TRACHEAL OBSTRUCTION. Rarely may give rise to sudden severe stridor and breathlessness but usually symptoms are more gradual in onset.

8. LYMPHANGITIS CARCINOMATOSA. Diffuse infiltration widely through the lungs is usually bilateral, but occasionally is unilateral and causes severe breathlessness.

DISTANT METASTASES. The commonest organs seen to be affected at autopsy are brain, bones, liver and adrenal glands.

Cervical Lymphadenopathy. The commonest sign of dissemination and occurs in 10–15 per cent of patients.

Cerebral Metastases present in 3–5 per cent of patients during life and should be suspected in patients presenting with personality change, hemiplegia or epilepsy.

Liver Metastases. Jaundice may occur without apparent enlargement of the liver but there is usually firm irregular rapid enlargement of the liver.

Bone Metastases. Especially affecting ribs, vertebrae and pelvis, give rise to painful, locally tender lesions.

NON-METASTATIC EXTRAPULMONARY MANIFESTATIONS
Endocrine Disturbances

i. *Hypercalcaemia:* Although it can be caused by widespread bony metastases it may occur alone when it is possible that a substance resembling parathormone is being produced by the tumour. This is commonest with squamous-cell carcinoma. Clinical features include polyuria and dehydration, muscular weakness, hyporeflexia, lethargy, drowsiness, anorexia, nausea, vomiting and constipation.

ii. *Inappropriate antidiuretic hormone (ADH) secretion:* Presents as anorexia, nausea and vomiting with restlessness, lethargy, mental confusion, irritability and weakness. Oat-cell carcinoma is the commonest type involved. The symptoms are due to water intoxication and hyponatraemia. This is recognized by a low serum sodium concentration and hypochloraemia with a normal or low serum potassium. The urine osmolarity is greater than the plasma osmolarity.

iii. *Cushing's syndrome:* Caused by the secretion of an ACTH-like polypeptide is not usually present long enough to cause overt physical signs. It presents as muscle weakness, lethargy and fatigue sometimes with severe depression. Gross dependent oedema may develop due to sodium retention and severe hypokalaemic alkalosis may develop. This syndrome is commonest with oat-cell carcinomas.

iv. *Melanosis:* Secretion of substances resembling melanocyte-stimulating hormone may cause hyperpigmentation.

v. *Gynaecomastia:* This may occur with the secretion of peptides resembling oestrogens or due to impairment of liver function preventing normal metabolization of natural oestrogens.

vi. *Carcinoid syndrome:* Oat-cell carcinomas may secrete 5-hydroxytryptophan causing diarrhoea, flushing and the other features of this syndrome.

vii. *Nephrotic syndrome:* May rarely occur with oat-cell carcinomas probably due to immune complex deposition on glomerular basement membrane. A specific antigen may be produced by the tumour or else antibody formation may develop in response to nuclear antigen released from tumour necrosis.

Neurological Disturbances. These are of unknown cause, often unrelated to metastases within the central nervous system, and are most commonly associated with oat-cell carcinoma. It is possible that substances are produced by the tumour that affect nervous tissue or else an autoimmune process may lead to degenerative changes. The neurological features often precede discovery of the primary tumour and they include the following:

1. DIFFUSE ENCEPHALOPATHY. This is characterized by anxiety or depression with loss of recent memory progressing to global dementia and disturbance of consciousness.
2. ENCEPHALOMYELITIS. This affects the brain stem and spinal cord and presents with ophthalmoplegia, pupillary changes and cerebellar disturbances.
3. SUBACUTE CEREBELLAR DEGENERATION. Typical signs of bilateral cerebellar disease may develop with vertigo, ataxia, dysarthria and progressive bulbar palsy. Dementia is common and there may also be muscular weakness and a peripheral neuropathy.
4. MYASTHENIC SYNDROME. This affects the proximal muscles with increased fatiguability but it differs from classic myasthenia gravis as the ocular and bulbar muscles are usually spared. The response to anticholinergic drugs is usually poor.
5. MYOPATHIC SYNDROME. This presents as proximal muscular weakness of subacute onset affecting the limb girdles and trunk. Clinical features include ptosis, bulbar paresis, loss of reflexes and peripheral neuropathy. These tend to fluctuate in severity and may show spontaneous remissions.
6. MOTOR NEURONE DISEASE. This is a rare pattern simulating motor neurone disease but with a more benign and prolonged course.
7. POLYMYOSITIS. This may present as widespread weakness and tenderness of muscles. When associated with skin changes it is termed dermatomyositis.

Skin Changes
1. DERMATOMYOSITIS. A lilac suffusion of the upper eye lids with a typical pink or purple raised rash over the face, forehead and cheeks. Sometimes the hands and fingers may be affected. There is usually an associated weakness and tenderness of the muscles of the hip and shoulder girdle.
2. ACANTHOSIS NIGRICANS. This presents as a brown elevated rash in the skin folds of the axillae, groins, and surrounding the mouth, umbilicus and anus.

Thrombophlebitis Migrans. Any type of bronchial carcinoma may be complicated by repeated peripheral venous thrombophlebitis poorly controlled by anticoagulant therapy. These often occur at unusual sites such as the neck, axillae or arms.

Finger Clubbing and Hypertrophic Pulmonary Osteoarthropathy. Finger clubbing occurs with about 15 per cent of bronchial carcinomas and may be present before the tumour is visible on chest X-ray. Sometimes it regresses following excision of the primary tumour. Less commonly an associated hypertrophic pulmonary osteoarthropathy develops with dull aching and swelling of the wrists and ankles. The ends of the radius or tibia show irregular subperiosteal new bone formation on X-ray.

Radiological Features. Always try to obtain previous X-rays for comparison. Common presentations are:

1. Rounded shadow often with an irregular border, this is probably the commonest finding.
2. Dense hilar mass: Can be caused by a tumour or associated hilar lymph-node enlargement. It usually has an irregular margin.
3. Localized ill-defined shadowing with the appearances of lobar pneumonia. Pneumonitis distal to proximal obstructing carcinoma is the usual cause.
4. Collapse of a lobe or segment. In adult smokers this appearance should always raise suspicion of an associated carcinoma.
5. Solitary cavitated lesion: This may resemble a lung abscess but fever is usually slight or absent.
6. Lymphangitis carcinomatosa. Diffuse spread of carcinoma through the lymphatics of the lungs causes shadowing which is usually asymmetrical. It is accompanied by severe breathlessness.

Tomography. Occasionally tomograms may be helpful in defining the features of a rounded opacity. It may also be useful if malignant cells have been found in sputum or there is haemoptysis and the plain chest X-ray appears normal. Although tomography is expensive and should not be a routine investigation it is valuable for detecting mediastinal infiltration by tumours.

Bronchography. This can be helpful for localizing endobronchial tumours not apparent on plain X-rays or tomographs.

Further Investigations

SPUTUM CYTOLOGY. The results obtained are dependent on the experience and interest of the cytopathologist. In good centres more than 80 per cent of bronchial carcinomas may be diagnosed from cytological specimens.

BRONCHOSCOPY. This is indicated for patients with abnormal chest X-rays where sputum examination has been negative and for patients with haemoptysis or malignant cells in the sputum where chest X-rays appear normal. Fibreoptic bronchoscopy has extended the range of exploration to subsegmental bronchi and with X-ray fluoroscopy biopsies can be taken from more peripheral lesions beyond the range of direct vision through the bronchoscope.

NEEDLE BIOPSY. Percutaneous needle biopsy of peripheral shadows with X-ray fluoroscopy often gives diagnostic histology when other methods fail.

PLEURAL ASPIRATION. Pleural effusions should always be aspirated for cytological examination of the fluid and sediment. A pleural biopsy may be obtained at the same time if an Abram's pleural biopsy punch is used.

MEDIASTINOSCOPY AND SCALENE NODE BIOPSY. Inspection of mediastinal structures by blunt dissection may provide tissue from mediastinal lymph glands for histological examination.

THORACOTOMY in an otherwise fit patient with an opacity on chest X-ray thoracotomy should be considered if other methods fail to give diagnostic histology.

Differential Diagnosis. In patients with cough, haemoptysis, finger clubbing or local chest X-ray abnormality the following must also be considered:

PNEUMONIA. Failure of radiographic improvement after 2–3 weeks of effective treatment should suggest a possible underlying bronchial carcinoma, especially in middle-aged smokers.

TUBERCULOSIS. Weight loss, night sweats, a history of contact with tuberculosis and mottled shadows in the upper lobes on chest X-ray favour a diagnosis of tuberculosis. Bronchial carcinoma may develop at the site of previous scarring from tuberculosis and may be associated with reactivation of the infection.

PULMONARY INFARCTION. There is usually a history of a predisposing factor such as immobilization or a recent operation but signs of venous thrombosis are often absent.

CHRONIC BRONCHITIS. Affected patients have an increased risk of bronchial carcinoma from cigarette smoking. Increased cough, haemoptysis, or the development of finger clubbing in a patient with chronic bronchitis should raise the suspicion of an underlying bronchial carcinoma.

'COIN' LESION ON CHEST X-RAY. Differentiation of a circumscribed bronchial carcinoma from other rounded opacities on chest X-ray may be difficult and extensive investigation may be necessary.

Treatment. The prognosis for bronchial carcinoma is poor and the majority of patients are dead within two years of the diagnosis being made and the 5-year survival rate without treatment is about 5 per cent. Patients with overt metastases are usually dead within a year. Where feasible, surgery is the treatment of choice as it offers a 25–30 per cent 5-year survival for patients with squamous-cell carcinoma suitable for resection. However, surgical resection is only feasible in 20–25 per cent of patients.

SURGERY. Lobectomy or pneumonectomy and occasionally segmental resection may be possible. There is no consensus yet of the extent of investigations necessary before proceeding to operation. Contraindications to surgery include evidence of metastatic infiltration of the liver, lymph nodes or bones, recurrent laryngeal nerve or phrenic nerve palsies and involvement of the brachial plexus or other structures. It is likely that preoperative assessment with liver and bone scans as well as mediastinoscopy should be regarded as essential.

Contraindications to Operation.

1. Age: Over the age of 60 the mortality rate is about 10 per cent for lobectomy and 20 per cent for pneumonectomy. Otherwise the operative mortality should be about 6 per cent.
2. Inadequate pulmonary function: If the FEV_1, or carbon monoxide transfer factor is reduced to 50 per cent or less of predicted values, operation will be impracticable.
3. Local extension of tumour or evidence of metastases are contraindications to surgery.

Palliative Surgery. May sometimes be considered in cases of Pancoast tumour with erosion of the brachial plexus or for severe haemoptysis.

RADIOTHERAPY

Radical Radiotherapy. The requirements are similar to those for surgery, i.e. that there is no evidence of extrathoracic spread. A malignant pleural effusion is a contraindication to radiotherapy. Hitherto, radiotherapy has been the treatment of choice for oat-cell carcinoma.

Palliative Radiotherapy. Should be reserved for the treatment of bone pain, severe haemoptysis or distressing breathlessness due to impending occlusion of the trachea or a major bronchus.

CHEMOTHERAPY. Numerous trials are in progress at present and it seems likely that treatment of oat-cell carcinomas will yield the best results. Adenocarcinomas and large cell tumours are insensitive to chemotherapy at present. For malignant pleural effusions reaccumulation following aspiration may be prevented by instillation of mustine hydrochloride, bleomycin or mepacrine into the pleural space after the fluid has been fully aspirated.

GENERAL TREATMENT. Treatment with antibiotics may control infection relieving breathlessness, cough and haemoptysis. Contact with patients should be maintained and the diagnosis should be discussed with those in whom there are indications that it would be helpful. The next of kin should always be fully informed. Diazepam and chlorpromazine may occasionally be necessary to allay anxiety in the terminal stages and the use of corticosteroids and opiates may ease suffering.

Prevention. Cigarette smoking is a major cause of carcinoma and vigorous attempts on the part of the medical and related professions must be continued in order that it may be eradicated.

BRONCHIAL ADENOMAS

These are the commonest benign neoplasms of the lung. Carcinoid tumours are the commonest type. The rare cylindromas are more likely to metastasize.

Pathology. They arise from bronchial mucous glands. Carcinoid tumours consist of well-differentiated small cuboidal cells while cylindromas are more pleomorphic in appearance.

Clinical Features. These are highly vascular tumours, so haemoptysis is a common early symptom. Cough due to bronchial irritation may be a presenting feature and obstruction of a bronchus may result in local wheezing and distal infection.

> CARCINOID SYNDROME. The secretion of serotonin, 5-hydroxytryptophan and bradykinin-like peptides causes flushing attacks associated with anxiety, tremulousness, fever, periorbital and facial oedema, lacrimation and salivation. Abnormalities of the valves of the left heart may develop. Osteogenic bone metastases are also common. Investigations should include assays for urinary 5-hydroxyindole acetic acid. Apparently benign carcinoid tumours may undergo malignant change.

Treatment. Bronchial cylindromas and carcinoid tumours should be resected by lobectomy combined with clearance of hilar lymph glands.

HAMARTOMA

These tumours are composed of various tissues normally occurring in the lungs but arranged in abnormal structures. They present after the age of 50 usually at the periphery of the lungs and are most commonly detected on routine chest X-rays as a 'coin' lesion with a smooth outline and 'popcorn' calcification. These are non-malignant tumours.

Arteriovenous Fistulae. These are rare vascular malformations causing a left-to-right pulmonary capillary shunt. They present with central cyanosis, breathlessness, finger clubbing and polycythaemia. There may be a systolic murmur audible over the fistula. Chest X-rays show a rounded opacity a few centimetres in diameter usually at the periphery of the lung. Thirty per cent of patients have hereditary telangiectasia.

METASTATIC MALIGNANT INVASION OF THE LUNGS

The lungs are commonly invaded by metastatic spread from tumours elsewhere and by the lymphomas.

Pulmonary Metastases. Spread to the lungs may be blood-borne as tumour emboli and by lymphatic spread from the thoracic duct. Metastases may be single or multiple. The commonest sites of origin of primary tumours metastasizing to lung in decreasing order of frequency are breast, stomach, large bowel, kidney, thyroid, bone and genital tract. Except where the metastases are very extensive or they cause lymphangitis carcinomatosa they do not usually cause symptoms. When symptoms do occur cough, breathlessness or chest pain are the commonest. Haemoptysis is uncommon because of the extra bronchial site of most metastases. Excision of solitary secondary deposits in the lung may be followed by freedom from recurrence for several years.

MALIGNANT LYMPHOMAS

Hodgkin's disease and other lymphomas most commonly invade the lungs by spread from mediastinal lymph glands but they may occasionally present with diffuse infiltrates or solitary opacities on chest X-ray without hilar gland enlargement. Tissue biopsy is usually necessary to establish the diagnosis.

MESOTHELIOMA

This tumour develops some 30–40 years after exposure to asbestos, especially the blue variety (crocidolite). A clear history of occupational exposure is not always obtainable and relatively brief exposure to contaminated clothing or atmospheric pollution near to asbestos works may be enough to predispose a patient to the risk of mesothelioma. A significant history is absent in about one-third of cases. Other signs of asbestos exposure, including pulmonary fibrosis, are often present on examination.

Clinical Presentation. The onset is usually insidious with dull aching pain and progressive breathlessness on exertion. Later, breathlessness may be present at rest due to increasing pleural involvement. There is often an associated pleural effusion.

Investigation. Chest X-rays show a large pleural shadow often in association with pulmonary fibrosis and calcified pleural plaques. Pleural fluid, often bloodstained, when examined will usually show abnormal cells.

Course and Treatment. The average survival is about 2 years from diagnosis. Surgery, radiotherapy and chemotherapy have not yet produced encouraging results. Death from ventilatory failure and intercurrent chest infection is usual.

Chapter 20

PULMONARY VASCULAR DISORDERS

Pulmonary Thrombo-embolic Diseases; Pulmonary Embolism; Chronic Thrombo-embolic Pulmonary Hypertension; Idiopathic Primary Pulmonary Hypertension; Arteriovenous Fistulae; Idiopathic Pulmonary Haemosiderosis; Goodpasture's Syndrome.

PULMONARY THROMBO-EMBOLIC DISEASES

Definitions. *Pulmonary embolism* usually refers to the impaction in the pulmonary arterial circulation of a venous thrombus from the systemic veins and *pulmonary infarction* is the pathological change which develops in the lung as a result of a pulmonary embolus.

Epidemiology. The true incidence of pulmonary embolism is unknown. Five per cent of routine autopsies show ante-mortem thrombus in the pulmonary veins. Of patients in hospital who develop pulmonary emboli about 50 per cent die of this cause. The sex distribution is equal and the incidence increases over the age of 45 years.

Pathogenesis. Most pulmonary emboli originate in the deep veins of the calves or ileofemoral veins. Other common sites of origin are the pelvic veins after childbirth and pelvic surgery. About 10 per cent arise from the right atrium in association with atrial fibrillation or mural thrombus following myocardial infarction. Uncommon non-thrombotic embolism may be caused by air, fat, malignant cells, amniotic fluid, parasites, endothelial vegetations and foreign material. These will not be dealt with in this section.

Venous thrombosis is encouraged by venous stasis, trauma to veins and coagulation abnormalities.

VENOUS STASIS. This is the most important factor.

Contributory causes include:

1. *Immobilization*: e.g. confinement to bed or chair.
2. *Low cardiac output*: e.g. heart failure or after acute myocardial infarction.
3. *Compression* of calf muscles.

Venous blood flow is diminished in ambulant patients with obesity, varicose veins and inactivity, e.g. during long journeys seated. In pregnancy mechanical obstruction of the inferior vena cava by the uterus and venous dilatation due to hormonal changes together with increases in fibrinogen and Factor VIII may encourage venous thrombosis. Hormonal factors may also be important in the puerperium and in women taking high-oestrogen oral contraceptives. In malignant disease, especially carcinoma of the pancreas, thrombo-embolism is common. Release of thromboplastins may be a causative factor.

VENOUS TRAUMA. Trauma to the lower limbs, especially fractures of the hip in the elderly, are a major cause of venous thrombosis. Local trauma to calf veins through recumbency during operations is an important contributory factor to the high incidence of venous thrombosis following surgery.

COAGULATION DEFECTS. Hypercoagulability of the blood occurs during recovery from trauma, surgery and childbirth and with thrombocythaemia, primary and secondary polycythaemia and following splenectomy.

Clinical Evidence of Venous Thrombosis. Overt symptoms and signs of venous thrombosis are absent in more than half the affected patients. Where present the following signs are helpful:

Swelling, warmth and tenderness of the calf or affected limb. Slight uni-lateral ankle oedema is easily overlooked. Pain on dorsiflexion of the foot (Homans's sign) may be present in about half the affected patients.

Tests to Confirm the Presence of Venous Thrombosis
1. ULTRASONICS using the Doppler technique. The ultrasonic probe is placed over a major vein proximal to the suspected thrombus. The limb is massaged and flow recorded in the vein is reduced if a thrombus is present.
2. ^{125}I FIBRINOGEN. This isotope is given by intravenous injection and uptake is measured over the limbs. Increased uptake may indi-cate fibrinogen being incorporated into fresh thrombus.
3. VENOGRAPHY. Radio-opaque contrast medium is injected into the foot to outline major venous occlusions.

Pathology
1. EMBOLUS. Pulmonary emboli are usually multiple and the lower lobes are most often affected. The majority are completely dispersed within 2 or 3 weeks but if repeated emboli occur organization, obliteration and distortion of vessels may lead to severe pulmonary arterial obstruction. Besides mechanical obstruction the release of vaso-active substances such as 5-hydroxytryptamine (serotonin) may also contribute to the increased pulmonary arterial pressure.
2. INFARCTION. With occlusion of a pulmonary artery congestion of the capillary bed and neighbouring alveoli follows but precap-illary anastomoses between bronchial and pulmonary vessels usually prevent necrosis of lung tissue. Pulmonary venous obstruction in mitral stenosis or left ventricular failure and occlusion of very large branches of the pulmonary artery predispose to pulmonary in-farction.

Clinical Features, Diagnosis and Management

MASSIVE PULMONARY EMBOLUS. *Symptoms*: sudden collapse or faintness, central chest pain, acute breathlessness. Pleuritic pain and haemoptysis occur in some cases. *Signs*: Pallor, slight cyanosis, sweating and sometimes transient loss of consciousness. Rapid feeble pulse, low blood pressure, pale cold peripheries. Raised JVP, gallop rhythm with third and fourth heart sounds. In most cases the diagnosis is obvious with circumstantial evidence such as a recent operation.

Differential Diagnosis

1. ACUTE MYOCARDIAL INFARCTION. Excessive breathlessness without pulmonary oedema favours pulmonary embolus. The ECG is often normal with pulmonary embolus but the presence of right bundle-branch block and T-wave inversion in leads V_1 to V_4 is helpful in making the diagnosis.
2. INTERNAL HAEMORRHAGE. The low JVP of haemorrhage contrasts with the high JVP of pulmonary embolus.
3. GRAM-NEGATIVE BACTERAEMIA. The JVP is usually low with peripheral vasodilatation.
4. CARDIAC TAMPONADE. The onset is more gradual with a paradoxical change in venous pressure. The heart shadow on chest X-ray will be enlarged.
5. AORTIC DISSECTION. The JVP is usually low and the aortic shadow will be widened on chest X-ray.
6. PNEUMOTHORAX. The breath sounds will be absent over the affected lung and the chest X-ray signs usually differentiate the two conditions.

Confirmatory Tests

1. CHEST X-RAY. There will be areas of reduced vascular markings and the pulmonary trunk may appear prominent.
2. ECG. A sinus tachycardia and low voltage complexes are common. The classic S_1 Q_3 T_3 pattern with T-wave inversion in the right precordial leads is unusual. Other occasional signs include right bundle-branch block, right axis deviation, a deep S wave in lead V_5 and P pulmonale due to right ventricular and atrial dilatation.
3. BLOOD GAS ANALYSIS. Will show hypoxaemia, hypocapnia and severe metabolic acidosis.
4. PULMONARY ANGIOGRAM. These are useful in doubtful cases to define the extent of the obstruction.

Treatment

1. EMERGENCY. Oxygen should be given by mask or endotracheal tube with external cardiac massage. An i.v. infusion of sodium

bicarbonate will correct the acidosis. Vasopressor drugs, e.g. isoprenaline, may be necessary to support the circulation.

2. FIBRINOLYTIC THERAPY. This should begin with streptokinase
600 000 units by i.v. injection followed by an i.v. infusion of
100 000 units per hour for 72 hours. Corticosteroids may reduce
the side effects of the treatment. Treatment is monitored by measuring the thrombin clotting time maintaining it at 2—4 times the
control value. Treatment is contraindicated with active peptic
ulceration, uncontrolled systemic hypertension, known bleeding
states, pregnancy or within 7—10 days of operation.

3. EMBOLECTOMY. This should be preceded by pulmonary angiogram to confirm the diagnosis. Mortality rates for emergency
embolectomy vary from 25 to 50 per cent.

4. ANTICOAGULANT TREATMENT with heparin is used after
embolectomy or streptokinase.

Prognosis. About 40 per cent of patients with acute massive pulmonary
embolus die within 10 minutes of the onset of symptoms, about 30 per
cent more survive 2 hours or more.

MEDIUM-SIZED PULMONARY EMBOLUS WITH PULMONARY INFARCTION

Symptoms. Sudden pleuritic pain, perhaps referred to the shoulder tip or
abdomen. Breathlessness with rapid shallow breathing. Haemoptysis occurs
in about half the patients. Cyanosis and slight jaundice may develop.

Signs. Moderate tachycardia, low grade fever, a pleural friction rub followed
by signs of a pleural effusion.

Investigations

1. CHEST X-RAY. May show linear shadows, a pleural effusion and
elevation of the hemidiaphragm on the affected side.

2. WBC. Polymorph leucocytosis of $15—20 \times 10^3/dl$. The ESR and
serum lactic dehydrogenase level may be raised. Arterial blood
analysis may show a low carbon dioxide tension with normal or low
arterial oxygen tension. Perfusion scans of the lungs will show
multiple areas of reduced uptake. Pulmonary angiography may
occasionally be indicated if the diagnosis remains in doubt.

Differential Diagnosis. This may be difficult because none of the signs are
unique to pulmonary embolism. Conditions to be excluded are lobar or
segmental pneumonia, bronchial carcinoma, postoperative collapse of the
lung, spontaneous pneumothorax and polyarteritis nodosa.

Treatment

1. Immediate: Relief of pain with opiates and administration of oxygen
for breathlessness.

2. Anticoagulation with heparin and then warfarin, continued for
   6–12 weeks.

Prognosis. Anticoagulants usually prevent the formation of new thrombus. The long-term prognosis depends on whether multiple emboli have obliterated much of the pulmonary circulation.

CHRONIC THROMBO-EMBOLIC PULMONARY HYPERTENSION

This is usually insidious in onset. Breathlessness is a prominent symptom, first present only on exertion but later at rest too. There may be no history of pleuritic pain or haemoptysis. Other features include syncope on exertion, angina pectoris from low cardiac output and sometimes persistent fever. Signs of right ventricular strain and pulmonary hypertension include giant 'a' waves in the JVP, a parasternal heave indicating right ventricular hypertrophy, a loud pulmonary second sound with reduced or absent splitting and right ventricular gallop rhythm caused by pulmonary hypertension.

Investigations
1. CHEST X-RAY. This may show prominence of the pulmonary trunk and the proximal pulmonary arteries with hypovascular or oligaemic peripheral lung fields.
2. ECG. Showing right axis deviation, P pulmonale and tall R waves in leads V_1 –V_2 with widespread T-wave inversion.
3. ARTERIAL BLOOD. Hypoxaemia and hypocapnia increasing with exercise.
4. EXERCISE TESTS. May reveal disproportionate hyperventilation and gas transfer indices (TLCO and KCO) may be reduced.
5. PERFUSION LUNG SCANS. These may show general reduction of the lung fields.
6. PULMONARY ARTERIOGRAPHY. This may be of limited value showing dilated proximal pulmonary arteries and rather slow pulmonary circulation.
7. CARDIAC CATHETERIZATION. This can be valuable to confirm the presence of pulmonary hypertension, especially on exercise and there will usually be elevation of the pulmonary capillary vein (wedge pressure). It will also exclude left heart disease.

Treatment. Long-term anticoagulation is the only available measure. The prognosis is good if pulmonary artery pressures are normal but a 50 per cent mortality within 5 years has been reported in patients with pulmonary hypertension.

IDIOPATHIC OR PRIMARY PULMONARY HYPERTENSION

There are probably two variants: (a) *Primary pulmonary hypertension*: This is commonest in young women, with widespread dilatation, medial hypertrophy and necrotizing arteritis affecting the medium-sized muscular pulmonary arteries; (b) *Pulmonary veno-occlusive disease*: This presents with obliteration of small and medium-sized pulmonary veins by fibrous proliferation of the media and intima.

Functional Disturbance. This consists of hyperventilation with increased dead space and ventilation–perfusion imbalance. Severe pulmonary hypertension may result.

Physical Signs. Are those of pulmonary hypertension with a giant 'a' wave in the JVP, parasternal right ventricular heave, right atrial and right ventricular gallop, a pan-systolic murmur of tricuspid regurgitation, a systolic ejection click and close splitting of the second sound. The ECG may show right axis deviation with right ventricular hypertrophy and strain.

Life expectancy for both forms of the disease is short; from diagnosis the average duration is 3 years.

Treatment of 'Classic' Primary Pulmonary Hypertension. Acetylcholine, tolazoline and hexamethonium have been used to reduce pulmonary vascular resistance but there is no evidence that they prolong survival. Anticoagulants and corticosteroids have been tried in veno-occlusive disease with little effect.

ARTERIOVENOUS FISTULAE

These are lobulated swellings connecting pulmonary arteries and veins, sometimes associated with haemorrhagic telangiectasia. Any part of the lung may be affected but they are commoner in the lower lobes. Small ones may pass unnoticed, but larger ones may cause a significant right-to-left shunt with cyanosis, polycythaemia and finger clubbing. A vascular murmur may be audible in about 50 per cent of cases. Treatment is by surgical correction as necessary. One important complication of this unusual condition is cerebral abscess due to the direct communication between right and left circulations allowing the passage of infected emboli from the veins.

IDIOPATHIC PULMONARY HAEMOSIDEROSIS

This rare condition is characterized by repeated intra-alveolar capillary haemorrhages and secondary iron-deficiency anaemia. It usually begins in childhood or early adult life and may be fatal, but complete recovery can occur.

Histology. The features include hyperplasia, degeneration and shedding of alveolar epithelial cells and localized alveolar capillary dilatation. Diffuse fibrosis may develop in chronic cases.

Symptoms. Chronic unproductive cough with tiredness, pallor and failure to thrive. Iron-deficiency anaemia develops from intermittent small haemoptyses. There are few physical signs, basal crepitations may be audible and about 25 per cent of patients develop finger clubbing and a similar proportion may show enlargement of the liver and spleen. A minority progress to cor pulmonale. Chest X-rays usually show multiple patchy shadows.

Diagnosis. This is confirmed by finding macrophages laden with haemosiderin in lung washings obtained by fibreoptic bronchoscopy or on lung biopsy material.

Treatment. Blood transfusion may be necessary for severe bleeding but the anaemia usually responds to treatment with iron. Corticosteroids are ineffective but immunosuppressive agents may be useful. Death may occur from massive haemoptysis. The average life expectancy from diagnosis is about 3 years.

GOODPASTURE'S SYNDROME

This is a combination of glomerulonephritis and intra-alveolar haemorrhage. It is commonest in young men with a male to female ratio of 4 : 1. Symptoms include cough and haemoptysis sufficient to cause anaemia. Progressive glomerulonephritis leading to renal failure is common. The lung and renal changes may precede each other or occur simultaneously. About half the cases develop from a prodromal influenza-like illness. Chest X-rays usually show widespread coarse mottling.

Histological Features. Antiglomerular basement membrane material has been identified in lung and renal tissue. Previously, treatment with corticosteroids and immunosuppressive drugs was ineffective but plasmapheresis may lead to improvement by removal of circulating immune complexes from plasma.

Chapter 21

THE LUNGS IN SOME SYSTEMIC DISEASES

Rheumatoid Disease; Systemic Lupus Erythematosus; Systemic Sclerosis; Polyarteritis Nodosa; Wegener's Granulomatosis; Lungs in Renal Disease; Histiocytosis X; Tuberous Sclerosis.

RHEUMATOID DISEASE

Lung changes in rheumatoid disease are generally commoner in men than women. They include:

1. Pleural adhesions, pleural thickening and pleural effusions which are commoner in men and may present with mild pleurisy and transient pleural effusions with a low glucose content and high lactic dehydrogenase content. Pleural biopsies usually show fibrosis and non-specific chronic inflammation.

2. Fibrosing alveolitis: Apart from the presence of arthritis there is little to differentiate this form of fibrosing alveolitis from others. The clinical and physiological features of this condition are unremarkable.

3. Rheumatoid nodules: These are much commoner in men and are associated with subcutaneous nodules which may pre-date the appearance of the arthritis. Histologically these nodules show central necrosis with plasma-cell infiltration and occasionally they may cavitate.

4. Rheumatoid pneumoconiosis (Caplan's nodules): These are small peripheral nodules (1–2 cm diameter) scattered throughout the lungs which develop in workers in rheumatoid disease who are exposed to coal dust, silica or asbestos. Rheumatoid factor is present in the serum in 80–90 per cent of cases. The lesions may pre-date the onset of arthritis and may cavitate.

5. Pulmonary infiltration with pleuropericarditis. This may present as pleural effusions and pericarditis with fever and breathlessness with little cough.

6. Pulmonary arterial obstruction with intimal hypertrophy and pulmonary hypertension. This usually occurs without an associated fibrosing alveolitis.

7. Rheumatoid laryngitis. Inflammation of the cricoarytenoid joints may lead to hoarseness and inspiratory stridor.

8. Respiratory infections. The incidence of bronchitis, obliterative bronchiolitis, bronchiectasis and pneumonia appears to be greater than normal in patients with rheumatoid arthritis and these conditions may often pre-date the onset of rheumatoid disease.

SYSTEMIC LUPUS ERYTHEMATOSUS (SLE)

This inflammatory connective-tissue disorder frequently involves the lungs. The histological features which are non-specific, include fibrinoid necrosis and cellular infiltration in the walls of blood vessels of any organ involved.

Pulmonary manifestations include:
1. Pleural effusions and pleural thickening, often with pleuritic pain.
2. Diffuse fibrosing alveolitis.
3. Pneumonic changes. Presenting as fever, breathlessness, cyanosis and tachycardia with diffuse radiological shadowing at the lung bases. Patchy local atelectasis or persistent consolidation may occur with features of cough, pleurisy and local crepitations.
4. 'Disappearing lung'. Many patients with SLE present with breathlessness, tachypnoea and chest pain without specific radiological abnormalities. Both lung function tests and chest X-rays show a progressive loss of lung volume.

Diagnosis. The diagnosis is made on the basis of the history and clinical findings and is confirmed by the presence of antinuclear antibodies (ANA) in serum. In some patients the ANA consists of antibodies to DNA (deoxyribonucleic acid). LE cells may be demonstrable in the blood of affected patients.

Treatment and Prognosis. Some patients respond to large doses of corticosteroids, e.g. prednisolone 40–80 mg daily. Azathioprine, chlorambucil or cyclophosphamide may suppress the disease in some patients and may be useful to replace part or all of the large doses of prednisolone which may otherwise be necessary to control the disease. The average survival from diagnosis was about 2 years before corticosteroids became available but now survival for 10–15 years is commonplace. Once a remission has been obtained treatment should be continued with maintenance doses of prednisolone for 6–12 months.

SYSTEMIC SCLEROSIS (Scleroderma)

This may affect the skin, gastrointestinal tract, lungs, heart and kidneys. The main respiratory symptoms are breathlessness and cough. The following lung manifestations may be seen:
1. Diffuse pulmonary fibrosis, similar to other types of fibrosing alveolitis. There is fibrosis with obliteration of alveoli and alveolar capillaries.
2. Restriction of chest wall movement due to progressive thickening and contraction of the skin of the trunk.
3. Inhalation pneumonia. Pneumonia and lung abscess may be caused by regurgitation of food and saliva because of oesophageal involvement. This is a common terminal event in systemic sclerosis.

The diagnosis is established by the presence of the features of the disease in other tissues including involvement of the skin and gastrointestinal tract.

Treatment. In some patients corticosteroids may be of benefit in doses similar to those employed for SLE but many patients fail to respond.

POLYARTERITIS NODOSA (PAN)

This rare disease, characterized by foci of necrotizing arteritis, involves the lungs in about a third of cases. Blood eosinophilia occurs in about 50 per cent of cases with lung involvement. Men are affected more often than women, and the disease is commoner over 40 years of age. The clinical manifestations include:

1. Low grade fever, weakness and weight loss.
2. Renal involvement, especially as acute glomerulonephritis with hypertension and renal failure.
3. Abdominal symptoms of pain, haematemesis and diarrhoea.
4. Involvement of the nervous system with cranial nerve lesions, polyneuritis, polymyositis or mononeuritis multiplex.
5. Muscle and joint pains.
6. Myocardial infarction, acute pericarditis and cardiac failure are all common.
7. Lung involvement with cough, haemoptysis, wheezing and features of pneumonia both on clinical examination and chest X-rays.

The lung manifestations commonly occur in patients with a previous history of bronchitis, asthma (usually severe) or pneumonia. Three lung lesions are recognized histologically: (a) necrotic areas presenting as cavitated nodules; (b) pulmonary infarcts; (c) bronchiectasis.

Clinical Presentation. Most cases present with a respiratory illness with fever, weight loss and general weakness and a high blood eosinophilia.

Investigations. A polymorph leucocytosis is common and an eosinophilia of 5×10^9/l or more occurs in half the cases. The ESR is usually very high. In a small minority of cases ANA and LE cells may be found.

Treatment. As for Wegener's granulomatosis.

WEGENER'S GRANULOMATOSIS

This is a disease associated with necrotizing granulomatous lesions of the respiratory tract with focal vasculitis and glomerulitis. It presents in middle age with an equal sex incidence. About two-thirds of cases are of insidious onset with nasal symptoms of rhinorrhoea, obstruction and pain with epistaxis.

Pulmonary manifestations include chronic cough, haemoptysis and pleurisy. Chest X-rays show rounded solitary or multiple opacities in about 50 per cent of cases and these may cavitate. The majority of patients undergo progressive deterioration within a few months, although a more benign form does occur. Treatment with immunosuppressive agents, including corticosteroids and azathioprine, may occasionally induce a remission. Plasmapheresis has recently been reported to produce striking improvement in some cases, perhaps through the removal of immune complexes from circulating blood.

LUNGS IN RENAL DISEASE

Pulmonary opacities on chest X-rays in patients with renal disease may be caused by pulmonary oedema, infections, emboli, lung damage from immune mechanisms, haemorrhage, calcification and the effects of drugs.

Pulmonary Oedema. Patients on chronic haemodialysis have been shown to have increased pulmonary capillary permeability and may develop opacities on chest X-ray from fluid accumulation within the lungs without overt heart failure.

Infections. In addition to common bacterial and viral infections, patients with renal disease, especially immunosuppressed, are particularly liable to infection with *Pneumocystis carinii* and *Cytomegalovirus* (*see* Chapter 15). Metastatic calcification of the lungs may develop in patients with chronic renal failure perhaps through injudicious vitamin D therapy.

Lung Function and Uraemia. Uraemic patients commonly develop a restrictive ventilatory defect (reduced FEV_1, FVC and TLC) with reduced gas transfer (TLCO and KCO).

HISTIOCYTOSIS X

Eosinophilic granuloma, Letterer–Siwe disease and Hand–Schüller–Christian disease.

These three conditions are related and are probably all variants of the same process. They are characterized by the presence of granulomatous tissue with plentiful cells resembling histiocytes. These lesions may affect many tissues including the lungs and bones.

Eosinophilic Granuloma. This may present with cough and breathlessness and about a third of patients develop a pneumothorax from rupture of cystic lesions within the lungs. The characteristic lesion is a greyish-white mass involving the lungs which progresses to honeycombing and more miliary shadowing on chest X-ray. As the disease advances widespread fibrosis develops. Pulmonary hypertension may result from involvement of pulmonary arteries.

Letterer—Siwe Disease. This affects infants and young children. A characteristic skin rash is present and the lungs are filled with multiple, small honeycomb cysts.

Hand—Schüller—Christian Disease. This presents with cavitating granulomatous lesions containing foamy histiocytes and lipid leading to widespread cavitation and fibrosis of the lungs.

Treatment. Corticosteroids in large doses may produce dramatic improvement, especially in Letterer—Siwe diseases.

TUBEROUS SCLEROSIS

This is another condition which presents with widespread honeycombing and fibrosis of the lungs. The extrapulmonary manifestations include adenoma sebaceum, subungual fibromas, kidney tumours and heart and bone lesions. The commonest pulmonary presentation is with a spontaneous pneumothorax from rupture of a cyst. Pleural effusions may also occur. Mental defect and epileptic fits caused by involvement of the CNS seem to be less common in patients with pulmonary involvement.

Chapter 22

MEDIASTINAL PROBLEMS

Mediastinal Masses; Mediastinal Emphysema; Acute Mediastinitis; Fibrosing Mediastinitis.

MEDIASTINAL MASSES (*Fig.* 24)

Although mediastinal masses may arise from a wide variety of tissues they may be grouped under three headings:

1. Cysts and primary neoplasms.
2. Lymph adenopathies.
3. Other space-occupying lesions.

General Manifestations of Mediastinal Masses. Whether benign or malignant mediastinal masses tend to enlarge and compress adjacent structures. *Benign cysts or tumours* may grow to large size but unless they arise in very confined spaces (e.g. thoracic inlet, intervertebral spaces) they give rise to few symptoms. They are usually clearly defined on chest X-rays. *Malignant tumours and aortic aneurysms* commonly cause early functional disturbances. The following are common: Invasion of the trachea with cough, breathlessness and stridor. Bronchial invasion causing cough and breathlessness. Oesophageal invasion or compression results in dysphagia. Superior vena caval obstruction will present as swelling and cyanosis of the face, neck and upper limbs with non-pulsatile distension of the neck veins. Pericardial invasion causes pericarditis and occasionally pericardial effusion

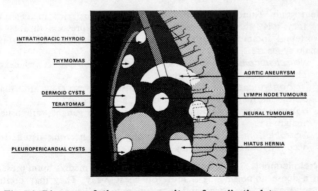

Fig. 24. Diagram of the common sites of mediastinal tumours on lateral chest X-ray.

with tamponade. Compression or invasion of the sympathetic trunk will give a Horner's syndrome with ptosis, myosis, anhydrosis and en-ophthalmos on the affected side. Phrenic nerve compression or invasion leads to paresis of the hemidiaphragm and sometimes persistent hiccups. Involvement of the left, or rarely the right, recurrent laryngeal nerve will cause hoarseness.

CYSTS AND PRIMARY NEOPLASMS

1. Bronchogenic and Enterogenous Cysts. These are derived from foregut tissue in the superior or middle mediastinum. They should be removed as they may become infected.

2. Pleuropericardial Cysts ('springwater cysts'). These arise in the cardio-phrenic angle, most commonly on the right. No treatment for this con-dition is needed.

3. Thymic Swellings. These arise behind the manubrium and may cause symptoms by compression of the trachea, bronchi or superior vena cava. *In infants* thymic hyperplasia is asymptomatic but may give a dramatic opacity in the superior mediastinum on chest X-ray. *In adults* thymic swelling may present as encapsulated cystic tumours containing calcified areas. Occasionally malignant change may occur but distant metastasis is uncommon. *Myasthenia gravis* occurs in association with about 40 per cent of benign or malignant thymic swellings and about 10 per cent of patients presenting with myasthenia have such swellings. Other conditions associated with thymic swelling include thyrotoxicosis, systemic lupus erythematosus and polymyositis.

4. Neurogenic Tumours. Usually found in the posterior mediastinum where they splay the ribs or cause spinal cord compression through the intervertebral foramina. Neurogenic tumours should always be removed. The main types are:
  a. *Neurolemmomas* of the sheath of Schwann on intercostal nerves. These are common and benign.
  b. *Neurofibromas* arise from the intercostal nerves. They are usually benign but may rarely undergo sarcomatous change.
  c. *Ganglioneuromas*. Arising from sympathetic ganglia, are usually benign.
  d. *Neuroblastomas*. Derived from sympathetic nervous tissue. Half occur in young infants. They are always malignant.

5. Teratodermoids. These usually lie in the anterior mediastinum present-ing as a dense homogeneous shadow on chest X-ray. They may contain both solid and cystic areas and may undergo malignant change. They should always be removed.

LYMPHADENOPATHIES

These are the commonest form of mediastinal mass and are of four main types.

1. Metastatic. Mediastinal lymphadenopathy is common with bronchogenic carcinoma and also with breast, gut and other tumours. Paratracheal node enlargement is common. Symptoms arise from local invasion of phrenic or recurrent laryngeal nerves and bronchi or trachea.

2. Tuberculosis. Paratracheal lymph-node enlargement forms part of the primary tuberculous complex in childhood. Paratracheal lymph-node enlargement is especially common in tuberculous infections of infants, erosion of the superior vena cava may lead to miliary spread. In adults, especially immigrants, unilateral or bilateral mediastinal lymph-node tuberculosis may present on chest X-ray.

3. Sarcoidosis. Bilateral, and occasionally unilateral, hilar lymph-node enlargement is the earliest and commonest thoracic manifestation of sarcoidosis. The paratracheal lymph nodes may also be enlarged so resembling the lymphomas on chest X-ray.

4. Lymphomas. Hodgkin's disease and other lymphoproliferative diseases may present with enlargement of the mediastinal lymph nodes. Low tuberculin sensitivity is common leading to confusion with sarcoidosis. Weight loss and fever are common.

OTHER SPACE-OCCUPYING LESIONS

1. Intrathoracic Thyroid. Either alone or extending from the gland in the neck; usually lies in the anterior mediastinum and may cause tracheal deviation and compression. Removal is advisable as haemorrhage into the gland may cause sudden swelling and acute tracheal compression.

2. Aortic Aneurysms. May arise anywhere along the thoracic aorta. On chest X-ray erosion of adjacent vertebral bodies with sparing of the intervertebral discs may be seen with aneurysms of the descending aorta. Linear calcification may be visible on X-ray and pulsation will be visible on screening.

3. Hiatus Hernia. Can present as a large cystic shadow in the lower part of the mediastinum, often seen in the PA chest X-ray as a fluid level within the heart shadow. Rarely hernias may occur through the foramina of Morgagni or Bochdalek in the anterior and posterior portions of the diaphragm respectively.

4. Achalasia of the Cardia. Dilatation of the oesophagus above the achalasia may appear as a posterior mediastinal mass on X-ray. An oesophageal pouch, usually in the upper part of the middle mediastinum, may be associated with achalasia or hiatus hernia.

5. Paravertebral Abscess. Pyogenic or tuberculous abscesses may resemble neurogenic tumours on chest X-ray. They may cause bony erosions.

6. Encysted Mediastinal Effusion. This may present as a shadow continuous with the heart shadow on the PA chest X-ray.

Investigation of Mediastinal Masses. Recognition of the site of the tumour on X-ray is all that is needed in some cases, e.g. pleuropericardial cysts. Tomography and screening may sometimes be necessary. Bronchoscopy, sputum cytology and mediastinoscopy are particularly valuable where lymph-node enlargement is present. Often thoracotomy is necessary to establish the diagnosis and exclude malignancy.

Treatment. Neural tumours, dermoid cysts, teratomas and thymomas should be resected because of the risks of malignant change. Intrathoracic thyroids should be resected to reduce the risk of tracheal compression following bleeding.

MEDIASTINAL EMPHYSEMA

Air may enter the mediastinum from rupture of alveoli, bronchus, the trachea or oesophagus or very occasionally from perforation of the bowel with passage of the air through the hiatus or other opening in the diaphragm.

Alveolar Rupture. May occur with severe asthma or emphysema or following violent coughing. The air tracks along the perivascular sheaths to the mediastinum and thence to the neck. There may be no associated pneumothorax.

Other Causes. Rupture of a bronchus, trachea or oesophagus may occur with foreign bodies, chest injuries or endoscopy. Occasionally oesophageal rupture may follow severe vomiting.

Clinical Features. If the air leak is large and especially if it is accompanied by food and gastrointestinal secretions it will cause severe pain and shock. Treatment with broad-spectrum antibiotics is indicated and gastrointestinal tears should be repaired when the mediastinum is debrided.

ACUTE MEDIASTINITIS

Causes
1. Oesophageal perforation is the commonest cause following endoscopy and laryngeal surgery.
2. Following suppurative lung infections, tuberculosis and osteomyelitis of the spine.

3. Haematogenous spread of infection from elsewhere.
4. Spread of subphrenic infection.

Clinical Features. Substernal pain, fever, rigors, dysphagia, pain radiating to neck and torticollis. A 'brassy' cough and breathlessness are common. Fever, cyanosis and restlessness are usual and there may be tenderness over the sternum.

Investigations. A chest X-ray may show mediastinal widening and displacement of the tracheal radiolucency on the lateral film. There may be mediastinal emphysema and a pleural effusion. The WBC usually shows a high polymorph leucocytosis.

Treatment. Should begin with broad-spectrum antibiotics in high doses, gastric suction and intravenous fluid replacement. Surgical drainage is necessary if persistent displacement of the trachea and oesophagus result from abscess formation.

FIBROSING MEDIASTINITIS

A rare disease of unknown aetiology but possibly related to Dupuytren's contracture, Peyronie's disease, Riedel's thyroiditis and pseudotumour of the orbit. Occasionally it is associated with retroperitoneal fibrosis, especially following methysergide treatment. Rarely it may follow infection with *Histoplasma capsulatum*.

Pathology. Macroscopically there is white, hard fibrous tissue encroaching on the superior vena cava and its branches but never invading the heart or lungs.

Clinical Features. Venous engorgement with swelling of the face and arms, later extension leads to obstruction of the oesophagus and trachea.

Investigations. Chest X-ray shows widening of the mediastinum. Inferior and superior vena cavagrams are necessary to delineate the obstruction and show the collateral circulation.

Treatment. Operation to relieve the pressure removing as much of the infiltrating mass as possible and by-pass grafts for the superior vena cava. Corticosteroids have proved unhelpful but some response to penicillamine has occurred in isolated cases.

Chapter 23

PLEURAL PROBLEMS

Spontaneous Pneumothorax; Pleural Effusion; Haemothorax; Chylothorax; Empyema.

SPONTANEOUS PNEUMOTHORAX

Definition. Pneumothorax is the presence of air in the pleural space with collapse of the associated lung resulting from penetrating injuries of the chest wall or traumatic rib fractures but more commonly from spontaneous rupture of the visceral pleura with leak of air from the lung.

Primary spontaneous pneumothorax without clinical evidence of underlying lung disease is common in young people being 5−8 times commoner in men than women and associated with tall stature. Primary spontaneous pneumothorax usually occurs in otherwise healthy individuals through rupture of small subpleural bullae, 1−2 cm in diameter, commonest at the apex of the lungs. Spontaneous pneumothorax is also common with connective-tissue disorders such as Marfan's syndrome and Ehlers−Danlos syndrome.

Secondary spontaneous pneumothorax is commonest in patients with chronic bronchitis and emphysema due to rupture of subpleural emphysema or bullae. Rarely a secondary pneumothorax may arise as a complication of pulmonary tuberculosis, severe asthma, pneumonia, lung abscess or bronchial carcinoma.

Pathogenesis. Contributory factors include rapid wide fluctuations in intrapulmonary pressure with increase in the pressure gradient across the pleural surface. Increase in pressure in subpleural air spaces from air trapping as a result of airways obstruction, the presence of large alveoli, lung cysts and bullae at the lung surface. When rupture occurs leakage of air will continue until the pressure gradient from lung to pleural space reaches zero. Rarely a valve mechanism may develop leading to a tension pneumothorax with progressive rise in intrapleural pressure causing mediastinal shift and compression of the opposite lung.

Three main classes of pneumothorax may be recognized:
1. CLOSED PNEUMOTHORAX. Where the hole in the visceral pleura closes spontaneously and the air in the pleural space is absorbed with re-expansion of the lung.
2. OPEN PNEUMOTHORAX. If the hole in the visceral pleura remains patent the lung will remain deflated and sometimes a direct communication between a bronchus and the pleural space forms a bronchopleural fistula.

3. TENSION PNEUMOTHORAX. Progressive increase in the intra-pleural pressure until it is above atmospheric pressure causes pro-gressive collapse of the affected lung, followed by shift of the mediastinal structures and compression of the contralateral lung. This is a fatal condition if not rapidly relieved.

Functional Abnormality. With a small pneumothorax functional impair-ment may be minimal but with larger pneumothoraces although perfusion of the affected lung continues, ventilation is reduced causing a large arteriovenous 'shunt' leading to arterial hypoxaemia. Later compensatory vasoconstriction develops with shift of perfusion to the remaining ventilated lung. In healthy adults with a moderate or large pneumothorax mild arterial hypoxaemia is common and exercise tolerance is reduced. The functional effects are greater if there is underlying lung disease. With a tension pneumothorax profound arterial hypoxaemia develops rapidly.

Clinical Features. The onset is usually sudden with breathlessness and sharp pleuritic pain, sometimes referred to shoulder tip. Occasionally a tight transthoracic pain may occur. An irritating persistent cough may occur and rarely there may be slight haemoptysis.

Clinical Signs. Breathlessness and tachycardia are common with cyanosis if there is underlying lung disease or a tension pneumothorax. A small pneumothorax may easily be overlooked but with a large pneumothorax chest movement is diminished. The affected hemithorax is resonant to percussion and breath sounds are diminished or absent. With a left pneumo-thorax cardiac dullness may be absent, while a right pneumothorax may reduce liver dullness. Occasionally a clicking sound in time with the heart beat may be audible with a left pneumothorax and may be accentuated if the patient leans forward.

Chest X-Ray. A PA chest X-ray will show lung collapsed towards the hilum with peripheral radiolucency due to the surrounding air in the pleural space. With a larger pneumothorax the mediastinum will be shifted to the opposite side and the hemidiaphragm on the affected side may be depressed. Small pneumothoraces at the apex are often difficult to detect on X-ray but a film taken on full expiration may be helpful as the size of the pneu-mothorax will be increased by the rise in intrapleural pressure on expiration. A large intrathoracic bulla may be difficult to distinguish from a pneumo-thorax on plain chest X-rays.

Differential Diagnosis. Other causes of chest pain and breathlessness to be considered include pneumonia, pulmonary infarction and acute myocardial infarction.

Course and Complications. If the defect in the visceral pleura closes the pneumothorax will resolve spontaneously because the partial pressure of gases in the pleural space is below that in venous blood. A pneumothorax in which 50 per cent collapse of the lung has occurred will take about 5–6 weeks to resolve spontaneously.

HAEMOPNEUMOTHORAX. Occasionally severe bleeding may occur, especially if there is a history of previous pneumothoraces with pleural adhesions. Rarely, *bilateral pneumothoraces* may occur simultaneously.

RECURRENT PNEUMOTHORAX is a common and annoying complication in both primary and secondary pneumothoraces.

TENSION PNEUMOTHORAX, if unrelieved, rapidly leads to death from peripheral circulatory failure and respiratory failure.

RESPIRATORY FAILURE is a particular problem, where there is underlying chronic lung disease.

PNEUMOMEDIASTINUM AND SUBCUTANEOUS EMPHYSEMA may result from an air leak into the interstitial tissues of the mediastinum and neck or around an intercostal drainage catheter.

PERSISTENT BRONCHOPLEURAL FISTULA AND EMPYEMA are rare complications, the latter most common when intercostal drainage has been used.

Treatment. The aims are re-expansion of the lung, prevention of recurrence of pneumothorax and return to normal activities.

1. *A small pneumothorax* with less than 30 per cent deflation in an otherwise healthy person should re-expand without interference. The patient may be ambulant but physical activities should be limited. Re-expansion can be accelerated by breathing high concentrations of oxygen (greater than 60 per cent) but the high flow rates needed are often uncomfortable for the patient.

2. *A large pneumothorax* should be treated by intercostal drainage to achieve rapid re-expansion and to avoid other complications.

INSERTION OF AN INTERCOSTAL DRAIN. Under local anaesthesia a large plastic or rubber catheter should be inserted through the 4th and 5th intercostal space, posterior to the anterior axillary line or through the second anterior intercostal space in the midclavicular line. Not more than 15 cm of the catheter should be introduced into the chest and it should be directed towards the apex. The catheter is connected to an underwater seal. Alternatively a Rubin flap-valve strapped to the chest may be used, this allows the patient to be ambulant. The chest is X-rayed daily to check the position of the lung and as soon as full expansion has occurred the tube should be clamped. If no deflation of lung occurs within 12–24 hours the tube is then removed. If the intercostal tube becomes blocked a fresh one should be inserted at a new site. When the lung fails to re-expand within 24 hours of insertion of the catheter, cautious suction may be applied to the drainage system. If the lung fails to re-expand with suction after 4–5 days, surgical seal of the lung defect should be undertaken.

PREVENTING RECURRENT PNEUMOTHORAX. An intercostal catheter may stimulate an inflammatory reaction in the pleura helping to prevent recurrence but this was commoner with the earlier red rubber tubes than the more modern non-irritant plastic type. Chemical or surgical pleurodesis is indicated if there has been a previous pneumothorax on the same side, especially if there have been contralateral pneumothoraces too.

1. *Chemical pleurodesis* is produced by instilling iodized talc or silver nitrate through a cannula into the pleural space. Lung function may be reduced by pleural fibrosis and this method should be reserved for patients with severe underlying lung disease unsuitable for surgery.

2. *Parietal pleurectomy* through a small thoracotomy is the treatment of choice for recurrent or chronic pneumothoraces. The parietal pleura is stripped but the diaphragmatic and mediastinal pleura are usually left intact. At operation small bullae or blebs on the surface of the lung can be ligated or resected and wedge resection of the lung apex is sometimes advocated for recurrent pneumothoraces but this is usually unnecessary.

Treatment of Complications

TENSION PNEUMOTHORAX is a dire medical emergency and should be relieved immediately by inserting any hollow needle through an intercostal space on the affected side. The needle can be replaced with an intercostal drain later.

MASSIVE HAEMOPNEUMOTHORAX necessitates open thoracotomy for haemostasis followed by removal of the intra-pleural haematoma.

PYOPNEUMOTHORAX should be drained through an intercostal catheter and a broad-spectrum antibiotic should be given.

SUBCUTANEOUS EMPHYSEMA AND MEDIASTINAL EMPHYSEMA without chest wall injuries can usually be avoided if tight sutures are not placed around the site of insertion of the intercostal catheter. No special measures are necessary as the emphysema resolves spontaneously.

PLEURAL EFFUSION

Fluid may accumulate in the pleural space by transudation or exudation in a wide variety of conditions.

Pathogenesis

In health there is a very thin film of fluid in the pleural space, amounting in total to 1 or 2 ml, which is produced by exudation of fluid from sub-pleural capillaries and absorbed into pleural lymphatics.

Pleural effusions may arise if any of the following occur:
1. Pulmonary capillary pressure is increased.
2. Pleural capillary permeability is increased by inflammation.
3. Pleural lymphatic absorption is decreased.
4. Plasma oncotic pressure is reduced.
5. With sodium retention.

Pleural effusions may be divided into exudates and transudates.

EXUDATES are caused by pleural inflammation, impaired lymphatic absorption or increased capillary permeability. A large effusion usually results with a high protein content (>3.5 g/dl) and high specific gravity (>1.015).

TRANSUDATES are caused by passive transudation of fluid into the pleural space by increase in pulmonary capillary pressure in congestive heart failure, loss of plasma oncotic pressure with hypoproteinaemia in nephrotic syndrome and cirrhosis of the liver. Transudates have a low protein content (<3.5 g/dl) and low specific gravity (<1.015).

Causes of transudates include congestive heart failure, nephrotic syndrome, cirrhosis, myxoedema and Meigs's syndrome.

Causes of exudates include malignant disease, bronchial carcinoma and metastatic carcinoma, pulmonary infarction, pneumonia, tuberculosis, collagen disorders especially rheumatoid arthritis and systemic lupus erythematosus.

Clinical Features
1. Breathlessness, prominent if the effusion is large.
2. Pleuritic pain occurs with inflammation of the pleura and may be referred to the shoulder tip if the diaphragmatic pleura is affected.

Physical Examination. A small pleural effusion may be undetectable, but if 500 ml or more of fluid are present chest wall movement is reduced, vocal fremitus is absent and percussion note, breath sounds and vocal resonance are reduced over the effusion. Occasionally bronchial breathing may be heard at the upper border of the effusion.

Investigations
CHEST X-RAY. The smallest effusion presents as obliteration of the costophrenic angle. With larger effusions a dense homogeneous opacity is visible in the lower part of the chest. The shadow extends higher at the chest margin because the sheet of fluid is here presenting a greater obstruction to the transmission of X-rays. Massive effusions may cause displacement of the mediastinum. If loculation occurs a semicircular opacity may be seen on the lateral chest wall, in the paravertebral gutter or in the interlobar fissure as an elliptical opacity. Films taken in the lateral decubitus position will show whether fluid is freely mobile in the pleural space.

Aspiration is essential as examination of fluid may reveal the diagnosis. The needle should be inserted under local anaesthesia into the midscapular line, one intercostal space below the point of maximal dullness to percussion. Care must be taken to prevent air entering the pleural space during aspiration. Not more than 1000 ml of fluid should be removed at any aspiration to avoid the risk of inducing re-expansion pulmonary oedema. The colour, specific gravity, protein and glucose content and cytology of the fluid should be noted and it should be cultured for micro-organisms, including mycobacteria. Pleural biopsy may be performed at the time of aspiration using an Abram's pleural punch biopsy but should not be attempted unless fluid is present.

Clinical Features and Treatment of Different Types of Pleural Effusion

1. POST-PNEUMONIC EFFUSION, usually small, secondary to bacterial pneumonia with a history of recent infection, pleuritic pain and fever. The fluid is clear or straw-coloured and usually sterile on culture if antibiotics have already been given. If cells are present polymorphs usually predominate.

2. PULMONARY INFARCTION. Small exudates are common with bloodstained or straw-coloured fluid. Aspiration is rarely necessary.

3. MALIGNANT
   a. *Bronchial Carcinoma.* Effusion is usually secondary to infection distal to a carcinoma. Less commonly the pleura may be involved by direct invasion with tumour.
   b. *Metastatic Carcinoma.* Especially from breast or bowel, less commonly, gives rise to a pleural effusion.
   c. *Pleural Mesothelioma.* Pleural effusion is a common feature of mesothelioma.
   In general malignant effusions reaccumulate rapidly after aspiration. The fluid which is usually bloodstained should be examined for malignant cells and pleural biopsy should be performed. Reaccumulation of malignant effusions may be prevented by instillation of thiotepa, bleomycin or mepacrine into the pleural space after removal of the fluid.

4. TUBERCULOSIS. Pleural effusions occur within 6 months of the onset of pulmonary tuberculosis and are rare in young children. Pleural biopsy should always be attempted in cases of suspected tuberculosis with effusion. The fluid is usually straw-coloured and contains lymphocytes. Culture is mandatory.

5. CONGESTIVE CARDIAC FAILURE. Small pleural transudate is common complication of severe left heart failure. Spontaneous resolution with diuretic therapy is usual and aspiration is not necessary.

6. COLLAGEN DISEASES. Pleural effusions are quite common,

especially with rheumatoid disease, where characteristically the clear fluid has a low glucose content (< 1.5 mmol/l) and a high lactic dehydrogenase content.

HAEMOTHORAX

Haemothorax usually results from traumatic injury but may complicate pneumothorax if pleural adhesions are ruptured. If large, the signs of the pleural fluid may be overshadowed by those of blood loss. Thoracotomy is often necessary to stop the bleeding.

CHYLOTHORAX

Chyle may accumulate in the pleural space from traumatic rupture of the thoracic duct or other large lymphatic channels. Invasion of other lymphatics by carcinoma, lymphoma and, more rarely, leiomyoma or leiomyofibromatosis may also cause chylous effusions. The diagnosis can be confirmed by giving the patient a lipophilic dye by mouth which will become visible in the pleural fluid.

EMPYEMA

Empyema or pus in the pleural space most commonly follows severe bacterial or tuberculous pneumonia or rupture of a lung abscess. It may also occur as a complication of chest injury, following surgery and as a result of oesophageal rupture, either spontaneous or after oesophagoscopy.

Clinical Features include a high swinging fever, profound constitutional upset and a high blood leucocytosis.

Management includes massive broad-spectrum antibiotic therapy. Occasionally pleural decortication becomes necessary later.

Dry pleurisy, i.e. pleural pain without signs of effusion, indicates inflammation of the pleura without radiological or clinical evidence of pleural effusion.

Chapter 24

COMMON DIAGNOSTIC PROBLEMS

Haemoptysis; Solitary Round Opacity on Chest X-ray; Diffuse Shadows on Chest X-ray; Lung Cavity.

HAEMOPTYSIS

Even a small haemoptysis merits thorough investigation as it may herald serious underlying disease. Check the history, be sure that blood has not come from vomiting or epistaxis. If haemoptysis is confirmed important factors are:

1. Age: tumours are more likely in older patients.
2. Quantity of blood.
3. Has it happened before?
4. Additional symptoms: chronic cough, breathlessness, wheeze, fever.

Possible causes to be considered are as follows:

1. *Short history with fever, cough and chest pain*
   a. Pneumonia (N.B. bronchial carcinoma or benign tumour may present with secondary pneumonia).
   b. Pulmonary infarction.
   c. Lung abscess.
   d. Inhaled foreign body – especially children.
   e. Acute or chronic bronchitis.
2. *Longer history with cough*
   a. Tuberculosis, especially in Asian immigrants.
   b. Bronchial carcinoma.
3. *History dating back to early life of cough with and without haemoptysis*
   a. Bronchiectasis.
   b. Hereditary haemorrhagic telangiectasia.
   c. Occasionally an aspergilloma may cause recurrent haemoptysis.
4. *Cardiac causes of haemoptysis*
   a. Mitral stenosis.
   b. Left ventricular failure.
5. *Other causes*
   a. Goodpasture's syndrome.
   b. Idiopathic pulmonary haemosiderosis.
   c. Bleeding diatheses.
   d. Anticoagulant therapy.
   Usually the history and examination are direct pointers.

Investigations

1. CHEST X-RAY IS MANDATORY: *If it is normal:*
   a. *In a young person,* if the haemoptysis is not repeated and there are no suspicious features in the history or examination, X-ray again at intervals of 1 and 3 months.
   b. *In older subjects* and smokers of all ages, fibreoptic bronchoscopy and sputum cytology are indicated.
2. OTHER INVESTIGATIONS
   Bronchography, especially in younger subjects, with chronic cough with purulent sputum where bronchiectasis is suspected but the plain chest X-ray is unhelpful. This may also reveal small endobronchial tumours and foreign bodies.
   Sputum smear and culture for mycobacteria either where the X-ray shadows suggest tuberculosis or with a clear X-ray in a young subject.
   Tuberculin test especially in the young who have not had BCG.
   No cause for haemoptysis found: In all patients with or without bronchoscopy the chest X-ray should be repeated in 4 weeks.
   RECURRENCE OF HAEMOPTYSIS AFTER BRONCHOSCOPY AND OTHER INVESTIGATIONS NEGATIVE: Repeat the bronchoscopy, consider the use of bronchography to search for intraluminal tumours.
   All patients with unexplained haemoptysis should be followed up for one year.

SOLITARY ROUND OPACITY ON CHEST X-RAY ('COIN' LESION)

Usually a chance finding on routine X-ray or because the patient presents with non-specific symptoms.

Common causes to be considered include:

1. Bronchial carcinoma.
2. Metastatic malignant disease.
3. Tuberculoma.
4. Benign tumour.
5. Hydatid cyst.
6. Pneumonia.
7. Lung abscess.
8. Pulmonary infarct.
9. Histoplasmosis.

Management

1. Try to obtain previous chest X-rays.
2. Chest X-ray features of help include:
   a. Margin of the shadow. If there is a hairline edge, it is likely to be a cyst or benign tumour.

    b. If calcification is not visible obtain tomographs. Calcification suggests tuberculoma or occasionally a hamartoma.

    c. An irregular edge to the shadow, although suggestive of carcinoma, may also occur with a tuberculoma and and other granulomas.

3. Clinical examination, search for enlargement of lymph nodes, liver and spleen and the presence of ascites. Feel the breasts or testes for nodules and swellings of tumours.

4. Tuberculin test: If negative, tuberculosis is unlikely. If it is strongly positive tuberculosis is a possibility.

5. Sputum cytology may be helpful.

6. Fibreoptic bronchoscopy and transbronchial biopsy with fluoroscopy may yield histological information.

7. Percutaneous needle biopsy under fluoroscopy may provide the histology. This is especially useful for more peripheral lesions.

8. Occult blood tests on faeces on three separate occasions indicates search for gastrointestinal malignant disease.

9. Barium enema and swallow may be indicated to exclude a gastrointestinal malignant primary lesion.

10. Intravenous pyelogram to exclude primary malignancy of the kidney.

If after these investigations no definite lead arises it is probably best to proceed to thoracotomy provided the patient is fit enough. Where operation is refused or not feasible the opacity should be assessed in follow-up chest X-rays. If it increases in size and the tuberculin test is positive a trial of antituberculous treatment may be given.

DIFFUSE SHADOWS ON CHEST X-RAY

Despite a large number of possible causes a combination of clinical data and a few relevant investigations usually lead to a firm diagnosis.

History. Details should be sought of past occupations, especially of dust exposure, hobbies and pets. Residence abroad is relevant because of possible mycotic infections. A history of dysphagia may suggest an aspiration or lipoid pneumonia. Symptoms of connective-tissue disease or malignant diseases. Rarely, recurrent haemoptysis may indicate primary or secondary pulmonary haemosiderosis. Details of all medicines taken during the preceding months or years.

    The patient with fever: miliary tuberculosis, bronchopneumonia and occasionally allergic alveolitis must all be considered.

    The symptom-free patient: possible causes include sarcoidosis, pneumoconioses, cryptogenic fibrosing alveolitis and rarely pulmonary alveolar proteinosis and microlithiasis.

    The patient with symptoms without fever: cough and weight loss rather than breathlessness suggest tuberculosis or diffuse pulmonary metastases.

If *breathlessness* is the prominent symptom possible causes to be considered are cryptogenic fibrosing alveolitis, allergic alveolitis, rheumatoid lung, honeycomb lung, haemosiderosis, diffuse pulmonary metastases and diffuse pulmonary lymphomatosis. Occasionally coal worker's pneumoconiosis uncomplicated by progressive massive fibrosis may present this way.

Details of Clinical Examination

SKIN LESIONS. Present in sarcoidosis, scleroderma, systemic lupus erythematosus and, rarely, sebaceous adenomas and subungual fibromas may occur with honeycomb lung.

EYE EXAMINATION. May show choroid tubercles in tuberculosis and uveitis in sarcoidosis.

JOINTS. Peripheral joints may be affected in rheumatoid arthritis or systemic lupus erythematosus.

HEART. Signs of right heart failure with right ventricular hypertrophy may be present in advanced pulmonary fibrosis from a variety of causes. In addition listen and look for signs of mitral stenosis which may accompany pulmonary haemosiderosis.

CHEST. Basal crepitations may be present with a wide variety of causes of diffuse lung shadows, but the presence of finger clubbing in addition suggests asbestosis, cryptogenic fibrosing alveolitis and rarely lymphangitis carcinomatosa.

LYMPH GLANDS, LIVER AND SPLEEN ENLARGEMENT. Occurs with lymphomas, leukaemia or malignant disease and less commonly sarcoidosis.

Investigations

1. CHEST X-RAY. Certain X-ray features are highly suggestive of particular conditions:
   a. *Hilar node enlargement* suggests tuberculosis, sarcoidosis, lymphoma or lymphangitis carcinomatosa.
   b. *The even micronodular pattern* of miliary tuberculosis is usually characteristic.
   c. *Bilateral mid-zone shadows,* in the absence of evidence of cardiac disease, suggests sarcoidosis.
   d. *Pleural plaques,* with or without calcification, are typical of asbestosis.
   e. *Very dense radio-opacities* suggest microlithiasis, alveolitis, varicella pneumonia or iron deposits.
   f. *Progressive massive fibrosis (PMF)* usually shows characteristic large cavitating opacities in the upper zones with other X-ray features of pneumoconiosis.
   g. *Other upper zone shadows* occur with tuberculosis or extrinsic alveolitis.

2. SPUTUM EXAMINATION. If infection is suspected proceed to bacteriological and mycological studies together with urine culture. Bone marrow and liver biopsies should be stained and cultured for acid-fast bacilli and other organisms. If malignant disease seems possible sputum cytology may be helpful.

3. BLOOD COUNT. This may be abnormal in leukaemias. A high eosinophilia may be present in polyarteritis nodosa, parasite infections and occasionally with asthma.

4. TUBERCULIN TEST. This can be helpful in differentiating between tuberculosis and sarcoidosis. If negative proceed to Kveim test, scalene node or lung biopsy.

5. IMMUNOLOGICAL INVESTIGATIONS. (i) Test for serum precipitins to *Micropolyspora faeni* and avian antigens may be of value. (ii) ANA and RF should be considered if systemic lupus erythematosus or rheumatoid disease seems likely. N.B. these may also be elevated in cryptogenic fibrosing alveolitis.

LUNG BIOPSY. Sometimes after full investigation it may not be possible to tell which of a number of possible diagnoses including tuberculosis, sarcoidosis, diffuse fibrosing alveolitis or metastatic malignant disease is most likely to be correct. Except in the very elderly or disabled, lung biopsy may be justified. The methods available include transbronchial biopsy with the fibreoptic bronchoscope under fluoroscopic control, percutaneous needle biopsy and open lung biopsy through a limited thoracotomy. The method chosen will depend on the age and fitness of the patient and the importance of obtaining histological evidence for treatment. It is usual to try transbronchial or percutaneous methods before thoracotomy.

LUNG CAVITY

In Britain the common causes of a cavity on chest X-ray are tuberculosis, lung abscess and bronchial carcinoma (a tumour may itself cavitate or cavitation may develop in infected lung distal to the carcinoma). With a history of *foreign travel* fungal infections such as histoplasmosis, coccidioidomycosis and blastomycosis must be considered as possible causes. Rarer causes of lung cavities include:

1. Metastatic tumour.
2. Infection of an emphysematous bulla or cyst.
3. Cavitation of progressive massive fibrosis in coal worker's pneumoconiosis.
4. Caplan's nodules (with rheumatoid arthritis and pneumoconiosis).
5. Breakdown of a rheumatoid necrobiotic nodule in the lung.
6. Ruptured hydatid cyst.
7. Amoebic abscess (especially in the lower zones).

Management

1. PATIENT FEBRILE AND ILL
   a. *Sputum.* Smear and culture for acid-fast bacilli, routine bacteriology and anerobic culture.
   b. *White Blood Count.* A high polymorphonuclear leucocytosis suggests a bacterial abscess. A relative or absolute lymphocytosis may indicate tuberculosis as the cause.
   c. *Blood Culture.* May sometimes reveal the causative organisms.
   d. *Sputum Cytology for Malignant Cells*
      Treatment should be started with a broad-spectrum antibiotic, e.g. ampicillin 0·5–1·0 g 6-hourly or amoxycillin 250 mg 8-hourly.

      If sputum on Gram stains or culture reveals organisms resistant to ampicillin and no clinical improvement has occurred the antibiotic therapy should be changed. If the fever resolves and serial chest X-rays show clearing of the shadow further investigation is unnecessary. If there is no resolution of the X-ray shadows and fever persists a trial of antituberculous chemotherapy may be indicated, avoiding rifampacin and streptomycin which have a broader spectrum of activity against non-mycobacteria. The best choice would be isoniazid and ethambutol.

      Fibreoptic Bronchoscopy. Indicated if there is no clinical improvement or the X-ray appearances are unchanged.

2. LUNG CAVITY UNCHANGING IN SIZE. Where bronchoscopy has been negative, acid-fast bacilli have not been identified and rare causes such as blastomycosis, hydatid cyst and amoebic abscess have been excluded, a thoracotomy may be indicated.

Chapter 25

DIAGNOSTIC PROCEDURES

Thoracocentesis; Pleural Biopsy; Transtracheal Aspiration; Lung Biopsy; Mediastinoscopy; Bronchoscopy.

THORACOCENTESIS

Diagnostic Thoracocentesis. The posterior chest wall medial to the scapula is the best site for puncture. With the patient leaning forward with his arms crossed, the soft tissues are infiltrated with local anaesthetic and a large-bore needle on a syringe is introduced firmly through the pleura with suction being applied to the syringe as the needle is advanced.

Therapeutic Thoracocentesis. With a large aspirating needle, three-way tap and a 50-ml syringe. It is often easier to use a 12- or 14-gauge radio-opaque intravenous cannula. The needle and cannula are introduced into the pleural cavity, the stylet and needle are then withdrawn and the catheter is left in the pleural space. The three-way tap and syringe can then be attached to the cannula and manipulated more easily.

COMPLICATIONS OF ASPIRATION

1. *High Negative Intrapleural Pressure.* This may develop if the lung is unable to re-expand freely. It causes tightness in the chest and coughing.
2. *Re-expansion Pulmonary Oedema.* This may occur if fluid or air is removed from the pleural space too quickly. It is best to limit the fluid removed to 750–1000 ml at each thoracocentesis. The features are a paroxysmal cough producing frothy oedema fluid and characteristic chest X-ray appearances of pulmonary oedema. The treatment is to reduce intrapleural pressure by allowing air to partly refill the pleural space.
3. *Air Embolism.* If the aspirating needle tears a superficial vein at the lung surface, air may be aspirated into the pulmonary venous system, most commonly causing transient cerebral symptoms. To avoid this the patient should be laid on his right side with the foot of the bed elevated.
4. *Empyema.* A rare complication of pleural aspiration if proper sterile methods are used.

PLEURAL BIOPSY

Abrams's Pleural Punch Biopsy. Should only be used if combined with thoracocentesis. When some fluid has been removed the soft tissues are incised with a scalpel and the Abrams's biopsy punch is introduced until the pleura is penetrated. The syringe is then attached to the inner tube and the fluid is aspirated. The notch on the outer cylinder is then located downwards, thus avoiding the neurovascular bundle of the rib above, and withdrawn until it snags against the parietal pleura. The inner cutting cylinder is then twisted sharply clockwise to take a biopsy. The whole instrument is removed and the biopsy specimen is flushed out with the fluid from the syringe. Useful pleural specimens are obtained in about 70 per cent of cases.

TRANSTRACHEAL ASPIRATION

In serious chest infections, especially in immune-deficient patients and those who have already been treated with antibiotics it is vital to try to obtain specimens of the pulmonary secretions uncontaminated by commensal organisms and debris from the mouth and oropharynx. This can be achieved by transtracheal aspiration with a needle or intravenous cannula inserted through the cricothyroid membrane with local anaesthesia of the skin.

LUNG BIOPSY

The available methods include percutaneous needle biopsy, high-speed trephine biopsy, transbronchial biopsy and thoracotomy. All methods may cause complications.

Percutaneous Needle Biopsy

1. TRU-CUT NEEDLE. This is less safe than some other methods but provides large specimens of diagnostic value in 80 per cent or more of cases of diffuse lung disease. Used with X-ray fluoroscopy it is possible to biopsy discrete peripheral opacities.
2. ASPIRATION NEEDLE BIOPSY. Simple aspiration with an 18-gauge lumbar puncture needle inserted through the skin under local anaesthesia can be very useful especially when infection is a likely cause of diffuse lung shadows. This method can also be used for discrete opacities if combined with X-ray fluoroscopy.

High-speed Trephine Biopsy. Large specimens of lung tissue can be obtained with diffuse lung diseases using the high-speed compressed air drill and trephine.

COMPLICATIONS OF NEEDLE BIOPSY. About 20 per cent of patients develop a pneumothorax which is usually asymptomatic and about one-quarter of these need an intercostal drain. Haemorrhage, rarely severe, occurs in about 10 per cent of patients and any haemoptysis is usually small and transient. Air embolism has been reported.

CONTRAINDICATIONS. Marked breathlessness, pulmonary hypertension, suspected vascular lesions, hydatid cysts, uncontrollable cough, and poor patient cooperation.

Transbronchial Lung Biopsy through Fibreoptic Bronchoscope. The biopsy forceps are advanced under fluoroscopic control until they meet resistance. They are then withdrawn about 1 cm and opened. The patient takes a deep inspiration, the forceps are then passed out until resistance is again met and when the patient has exhaled the forceps are closed and the enclosed piece of lung is avulsed. This method is invaluable for the diagnosis of sarcoidosis. With discrete lesions good results are obtained provided that they can be entered from an airway. In other diffuse diseases the small tissue samples provided by this method may not be sufficiently representative to form a definitive basis for treatment. The incidence of complications is less than with other methods.

Thoracotomy. Through a lateral or anterolateral limited incision. Persistent pain may be a problem but the postoperative mortality should be less than 0·5 per cent. The specimens obtained should be adequate for all purposes.

MEDIASTINOSCOPY

A mediastinoscope is inserted through an incision in the suprasternal notch, passed downwards through the pretracheal fascia to the upper mediastinum. By this means mediastinal lymph glands may be biopsied. The success rate naturally varies with the experience and enthusiasm of the surgeon.

BRONCHOSCOPY

The flexible fibreoptic bronchoscope is a major advance in the diagnostic facilities available for the investigation of pulmonary diseases. Because it can be used under local anaesthesia with minimal discomfort to the patient and can reach much more of the bronchial tree it has largely superseded the rigid instruments. Although the biopsy specimens obtained with the fibrescope are very small, advances in histological methods have ensured that the diagnostic yield is not less than with the rigid instrument but the latter is still best for removal of foreign bodies or of copious secretions. Fibrescopes are 4—6 mm in external diameter and can usually inspect the second or third generation of subsegmental bronchi. An additional advantage is the use of a side-viewing device allowing a second observer to watch. Small biopsy specimens can be taken from visible lesions, bronchial brushings may also be obtained and by combination with X-ray fluoroscopy biopsies from peripheral lesions beyond the field of direct vision may be obtained with the flexible biopsy forceps provided. The morbidity rate is low and mortality is rare. In addition the fibreoptic bronchoscope is being used for procedures including lobar and segmental gas flow studies and to harvest pulmonary macrophages and lymphocytes by lavage. The scope of the instrument has hardly begun to be explored.

A GLOSSARY OF TERMS

Lung Volumes (*see Fig.* 12, p. 39)

TLC, total lung capacity, the volume of gas in the chest at maximum inspiration.

VC, vital capacity, the maximum volume of gas which can be expired after a maximum inspiration.

FRC, functional residual capacity, the gas remaining in the lungs after a quiet expiration.

V_T, tidal volume, the volume of gas inspired or expired with each breath.

ERV, expiratory reserve volume, the volume of gas which can be expired by voluntary effort from FRC.

IRV, inspiratory reserve volume, the volume of gas which can be expired by voluntary effort from FRC.

IRV, inspiratory reserve volume, the volume of gas which can be inspired by maximum voluntary effort in addition to the tidal volume.

RV, residual volume, the volume of gas remaining in the lungs after maximum expiration.

IC, inspiratory capacity, the maximum volume of gas which can be inspired from the resting expiratory level (i.e. FRC).

TLC = RV + VC = FRC + IC.

RV = FRC − ERV.

IC = TLC − ERV.

PEFR, peak expiratory flow rate, the maximum flow over 10 milliseconds at the beginning of expiration with maximum effort after maximum inspiration (i.e. TLC).

FEV_1, forced expired volume in 1 second, the volume expired in the first second of a maximal expiration from full inspiration (i.e. TLC).

MMF 50, flow rate measured from the maximum expiratory flow volume, (MEFV) recording, when 50 per cent of the vital capacity has been expired.

MMF 75, flow rate measured from the MEFR curve when 75 per cent of the vital capacity has been expired.

PaO_2, partial pressure of oxygen in arterial blood.

$PaCO_2$, partial pressure of carbon dioxide in arterial blood.

TLCO, transfer factor for carbon monoxide, measured as quantity of gas transferred in unit time per unit difference in partial pressure between gas in the alveoli and in the mean capillary blood.

VA, alveolar volume, the lung volume calculated by a single breath helium-mixing method, used in calculation of TLCO and KCO.

KCO, diffusion coefficient for carbon monoxide, or gas transfer per unit volume of lung, i.e. TLCO corrected for lung volume, $KCO = TLCO/_{VA}$.

Trapped gas, the amount of gas in the lung which is poorly ventilated. It is calculated by subtracting a single breath estimate of lung volume (i.e. helium dilution) VA from plethysmographic estimate of TLC, i.e. trapped gas = TLC − VA.

BIBLIOGRAPHY

GENERAL

Crofton J. and Douglas A. (1975) *Respiratory Diseases*, 2nd ed. Oxford, Blackwell.

Edge J. R. (1970) *Lectures in Chest Medicine*. London, Staples.

Forjacs P. (1978) *Lung Sounds*. London, Baillière Tindall.

Fraser R. G. and Pare G. A. P. (1978) *Diagnosis of Diseases of the Chest*, 2nd ed. Philadelphia, Saunders.

Lane D. J. (ed.) (1976) *Tutorials in Post-Graduate Medicine — Respiratory Disease*. London, Heinemann.

Lillington G. A. and Jamplis (1977) *A Diagnostic Approach to Chest Diseases; Differential Diagnosis based on Roentgenographic Patterns*. Baltimore, Williams & Wilkins.

Murray J. F. (1976) *The Normal Lung: The Basis for Diagnosis and Treatment of Pulmonary Disease*. Philadelphia, Saunders.

Stretton T. B. (ed.) (1976) *Recent Advances in Respiratory Medicine*. Edinburgh, Churchill Livingstone.

Macklem P. T. and Permuitt S. (1979) *The Lung in Transmission from Health to Disease*. New York, Marcel Dekker.

RADIOLOGY

Simon G. (1978) *Principles of Chest X-Ray Diagnosis*, 4th ed. London, Butterworths.

Squire L. F., Colicae W. M. and Strutynsky N. (1970) *Exercises in Diagnostic Radiology, 1. The Chest*. Philadelphia, Saunders.

RESPIRATORY FUNCTION

Bates D. V., Maclem P. T. and Christie R. V. (1971) *Respiratory Function in Disease*, 2nd ed. Philadelphia, Saunders.

Campbell E. J. M., Dickinson C. J. and Slater J. D. E. H. (1974) *Clinical Physiology*, 4th ed. Oxford, Blackwell.

Campbell E. J. M., Agostoni E. and Newsom-Davies J. (1970) *The Respiratory Muscles*. London, Lloyd-Luke.

Comroe J. H. (1974) *Physiology of Respiration*, 2nd ed. Chicago, Year Book.

Cotes J. E. (1975) *Lung Function Assessment and Application in Medicine*, 3rd ed. Oxford, Blackwell.

McHardy J. G. R., Shirling D. and Passmore R. (1967) *Basic Techniques in Human Metabolism and Respiration*. Oxford, Blackwell.

West J. B. (1970) *Ventilation, Blood Flow and Gas Exchange*, 2nd ed. Oxford, Blackwell.

West J. B. (1974) *Respiratory Physiology – The Essentials*. Oxford, Blackwell.

West J. B. (1977) *Pulmonary Patho-physiology – The Essentials*. Oxford, Blackwell.

CIRCULATION AND PATHOLOGY

Fishman A. P. and Hechte H. H. (1969) *The Pulmonary Circulation and Interstitial Space*. Chicago, University of Chicago.

Harris P. and Heath D. (1978) *The Human Pulmonary Circulation*, 2nd ed. London, Livingstone.

Spencer H. (1977) *Pathology of the Lung*, 3rd ed. Oxford, Pergamon.

BRONCHOSCOPY

Ikeda S. (1974) *Atlas of Flexible Bronchofiberoscopy*. University Park Press, Baltimore and London.

Sackner, M. A. (1975) Bronchofibreoscopy – state of the art. *Am. Rev. Respir. Dis.* III, 62.

Stradling P. (1968) *Diagnostic Bronchoscopy*. London, Livingstone.

Zavala D. C. (1978) *Flexible Fibreoptic Bronchoscopy – A Training Handbook*. Iowa, University of Iowa Press.

RESPIRATORY INFECTIONS

Garrod L. P., Lambert H. P. and O'Grady F. (1973) *Antibiotic and Chemotherapy*. Edinburgh, Churchill Livingstone.

Jackson G. G. and Muldoon R. L. (1975) *Viruses causing Common Respiratory Infections in Man*. Chicago, University of Chicago Press.

Knight V. (1973) *Viral and Mycoplasmal Infection of the Respiratory Tract*. Philadelphia, Lea & Febiger.

May J. R. (1972) *The Chemotherapy of Chronic Bronchitis and Allied Disorders*, 2nd ed. London, English Universities Press.

Stuart-Harris C. H. and Schild G. C. (1976) *Influenza: The Viruses and the Diseases*. London, Arnold.

Tyrrell D. A. J. (1965) *Common Colds and Related Diseases*. London, Arnold.

CHRONIC BRONCHITIS AND EMPHYSEMA

Bates D. V. (1968) Chronic bronchitis and emphysema. *New Engl. J. Med.* 278, 546 and 600.

Fletcher C., Peto R., Tinker C. and Spizer F. E. (1976) *The Natural History of Chronic Bronchitis and Emphysema.* Oxford, Oxford University Press.
Lambert P. M. and Reid D. D. (1970) Smoking, air pollution and bronchitis in Britain. *Lancet* 1, 853.
Reid, Lynne (1967) *Pathology of Emphysema.* London, Lloyd-Luke.
Royal College of Physicians (1971) *Smoking and Health Now.* London, Pitman.
Petty T. L. (1978) *Chronic Obstructive Pulmonary Disease.* New York, Marcel Dekker.
Sykes M. K., McNicol M. W. and Campbell E. J. M. (1969) *Respiratory Failure.* Oxford, Blackwell.

ASTHMA

Austen K. F. and Lichtenstein L. M. (ed.) (1973) *Asthma—Physiology, Immuno-pharmacology and Treatment.* New York, Academic Press.
CIBA Foundation Guest Symposium (1971) *Identification of Asthma.* Edinburgh, Churchill Livingstone.
Clark T. J. H. and Godfrey S. (ed.) (1977) *Asthma.* London, Chapman & Hall.
Jones R. S. (1976) *Asthma in Children.* London, Arnold.
Stein M. (ed.) (1975) *New Directions in Asthma.* Illinois, American College of Chest Physicians.
Weiss E. B. (ed.) (1978) *Status Asthmaticus.* Baltimore, University Park Press.
Weiss E. and Segal W. (ed.) (1977) *Bronchial Asthma: Mechanisms and Therapeutics.* Boston, Little Brown.

CARCINOMA OF THE BRONCHUS

Deely T. J. (ed.) (1971) *Carcinoma of the Bronchus.* London, Butterworth.
Doll P. and Peto R. (1976) Mortality in relation to smoking: 20 years observations on male British doctors. *Br. Med. J.* 2, 1525.
Geddes D. M. (1979) The natural history of lung cancer: a review based on rates of tumour growth. *Br. J. Dis. Chest* 73, 1.

OCCUPATIONAL LUNG DISEASES

Morgan W. K. C. and Seaton W. A. (1975) *Occupational Lung Diseases.* Philadelphia, Saunders.
Muir D. C. F. (ed.) (1972) *Clinical Aspects of Inhaled Particles.* London, Heinemann.
Parkes W. R. (1974) *Occupational Lung Disorders.* London, Butterworth.

Pepys J. (1969) Hypersensitivity diseases of the lungs due to fungi and organic dusts. *Monogr. Allergy* Basle, Karger.

DIFFUSE LUNG DISEASES ETC.

Livingstone J. L., Lewis J. G., Reid L. and Jefferson K. (1964) Diffuse interstitial pulmonary fibrosis. *Q. J. Med.* **33**, 71.

Scadding J. G. (1974) Diffuse pulmonary alveolar fibrosis. *Thorax* **29**, 271.

Scadding J. G. and Hinson K. F. (1967) Diffuse fibrosing alveolitis (diffuse interstitial fibrosis of the lung). Correlation of histology at biopsy with prognosis. *Thorax* **22**, 291.

Turner-Warwick M. (1974) A perspective view of pulmonary fibrosis. *Br. Med. J.* **2**, 371.

SARCOIDOSIS

Mitchell D. N. and Scadding J. G. (1974) State of the Art: Sarcoidosis, *Am. Rev. Respir. Dis.* **110**, 774.

Scadding J. G. (1967) *Sarcoidosis.* London, Eyre & Spottiswood.

CONNECTIVE-TISSUE DISEASES

Hughes G. R. V. (1974) Systemic lupus erythematosus. *Br. J. Hosp. Med.* **12**, 309.

Rose G. A. and Spencer H. (1957) Polyarteritis nodosa. *Q. J. Med.* **26**, 43.

Rubin E. H. (1967) Rheumatoid lung. *N.Y. State J. Med.* **67**, 2014.

Turner-Warwick M. E. (1969) Rheumatoid arthritis, rheumatoid factors in lung disease. *Br. J. Hosp. Med.* **2**, 507.

Turner-Warwick M. E. (1978) *Immunology of the Lung.* London, Arnold.

INDEX